THE WORLD
BEAUTY BOOK

THE WORLD BEAUTY BOOK

How We Can All Look
and Feel Wonderful Using
the Natural Beauty Secrets of
Women of Color

JESSICA B. HARRIS

HarperSanFrancisco
An Imprint of HarperCollins*Publishers*

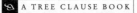
A TREE CLAUSE BOOK

HarperSanFrancisco and the author, in association with The
Basic Foundation, a not-for-profit organization whose
primary mission is reforestation, will facilitate the planting of two
trees for every one tree used in the manufacture of this book.

FIRST EDITION
Book design by Mauna Eichner
Set in Monotype Bulmer

Library of Congress Cataloging-in-Publication Data
Harris, Jessica B.
The world beauty book : how we can all look
and feel wonderful using the natural beauty secrets of
women of color / Jessica Harris.
p.   cm.
Includes bibliographical references and index.
ISBN 0–06–251092–4 (pbk.)
1. Beauty, Personal.   2. Minority women—Health and hygiene.
I. Title
RA778.H247   1995   95–6010
646.7'046—dc20   CIP

95 96 97 98 99 ❖ RRD(H) 10 9 8 7 6 5 4 3 2 1

*To all of the women of the world who enabled
me to see the beauty in me, by showing me
the beauty in them—particularly my
mother, Rhoda Alease Jones Harris.*

CONTENTS

Acknowledgments

THE LIST OF THANKS for a book such as this can run as long as the credits on a Cecil B. DeMille movie. Rather than attempt to list each and every person by name I shall simply say that thanks are owed to all of the members of my international circle of women/friends—you know who you are whether your name turns up in these pages or not. I depend on you all. By playing every role from chauffeur to griot, from priestess to herbalist, from mother confessor to cosmetician, you all have enabled me to sing our song with what I hope is a clear, true voice.

I must also thank the testosterone side of my international family. They too aided me in my quest, reminding me of the secrets of their mothers, suggesting others with whom I should speak, and understanding and enjoying my efforts to capture the elusive butterfly of our history.

Thanks are also due my agent, Carole Abel, who got the idea for this book when I first mentioned it to her over ten years ago. At Harper San Francisco, I must thank Barbara Moulton, my first editor, who acquired the text, and Lisa Bach, who worked with me to transform it into the book you have in your hands.

Finally, thanks are due to my mother, the living example of the timelessness of true beauty in my own life, and to the African Orișa, Christian God, Native American Life Forces, and Creative Spirits of my known and unknown ancestors who allow me to get up each morning and try to write. May this book honor them.

THE WORLD
BEAUTY BOOK

INTRODUCTION

FOR MILLENNIA, women have been searching for ways to enhance their appearance. We have looked everywhere, from nature to chemistry. Now, as the twentieth century draws to a close, we are discovering new places to look—within ourselves and at other women in the world around us.

This book grows out of my observations of and discussions with women around the world who have become my friends and my guides as I have traveled and lived with them for over four decades. While women of European descent have their own beauty rituals, the women who offer a glimpse into their lives in this book are women not usually heard from. These women, who have spent their lives on the margins of Western history, are unsung heroines who have kept the traditional fires of their cultures burning.

The women you will meet in these pages come from such places around the world as Senegal and Mexico, India and Haiti, Brazil and Benin, Guyana and China. Others are from right here: Native American and African American women with the secrets of their grandmothers and great-grandmothers. They are descendants of princesses and laborers, queens and commoners, empresses and slaves. Their skins may be alabaster white, eggplant black, or any color in between. They may live in mud huts or high-rise apartments, but they all share one thing. They all use the traditional beauty secrets they learned from friends and family.

These are women who use the old ways to enhance their looks—women who go to the nearest shrub or grass to provide color for their lips or a fragrance for their bath, who call their old aunt to find out about a rinse for their hair, or who visit the local herbalist for a tea to rid themselves of menstrual cramps. Many of their beauty rituals are at the origin of some of today's cosmetics. In this book, though, rather than using adaptations, or adulterated modern versions, we go back to the source, to the women themselves. They tell us about their ways of beauty in their own words.

The book is divided into eight chapters, which cover beauty from the inside out. The first chapter recounts the history of non-Western beauty and the story of how I gathered much of the information. Chapter 2 presents the life stages of beauty and discusses how to find yourself and be comfortable in each one. The following chapters look at hair, faces, and bodies. Recipes abound and speak of everything from dry shampoos and natural hair rinses to soothing soaks and care for the hands and feet. These chapters are the place to look for facial scrubs using cornmeal and avocados, salt rubs to make your body glow, sage breath fresheners, and hot oil treatments to help damaged hair.

Shocking pink silks, brilliant *kentes,* and sensuous turquoise brocades, the ethnic dressing of non-Western women, have made us birds of paradise in the world of fashion. In chapter 6, you will learn how to use elements of ethnic dressing to create your own fashion look, one that may speak to a culture that you admire or one that speaks of your own origins. In the same chapter, you will also learn about fragrances and how non-Western women use them to their beauty advantage. Special secrets shared between girlfriends, mothers, and daughters are the focus of chapter 7, which offers teas for relieving menstrual cramps, suggestions for cold cures, and a peek at some aphrodisiacs. The final chapter moves from you to your environment and shows you how to enhance your living space, your work space, and your life.

Each chapter offers concrete suggestions, with recipes and instructions on how to enhance yourself and your life using the beauty secrets of the worldwide sisterhood of non-Western women of color. A listing of suggested books gives those who wish to read more a place to begin, while a guide to mail-order sources enables you to find the occasional ingredient that may not turn up in your kitchen cupboard, at your health-food shop, or at your local herbalist.

What you hold in your hands is a passport to another world. Think of it as a personal telephone book filled with the numbers of girlfriends from around the world who have beauty suggestions to offer you. Read the book straight through, or pick it up and glance through sections as the need occurs. You simply have to open the book, turn to a chapter, and select a friend with whom to speak. The women will take it from there.

☙

Chapter 1

BEAUTY THROUGH THE AGES

Look Back in Time to Learn
Natural Beauty Secrets

ROM THE TIME of the earliest explorations, the Western world has been fascinated by women of color, women of the exotic world. The swish of an Indian silk sari, the sight of a delicate Asian woman in a Vietnamese *ao dai,* a glimpse of an African woman-child with a frightened fawn face, the sultry walk of a Latina, and the burnished radiance of Native American women have set imaginations on fire, sent more than one Western man on flights of erotic fantasy, and inspired reactions ranging from rage to envy to emulation. The beauty of women of color is potent indeed. Traditional ideas of beauty, beauty secrets, and ways of womanhood are ongoing secrets whose origins are lost in time.

No one knows how long cosmetics have been used, but the complex Neolithic cave paintings at Tassili n'Ajjer, Algeria, show that body decoration and adornment go back millennia and more than likely predate clothing. It is not difficult to imagine a prehistoric young woman dipping her fingers into a container filled with the same pigment that created the cave paintings, and adding a little touch here and there to "freshen up" her body paint.

The earliest beauty secrets were deeply ingrained in people's daily lives. While body painting and adornment may seem ornamental to us, they have always been part of a complex system that integrates ritual and medicine with a human desire for adornment. A woman's body paint may have signaled her social status, her physical prowess, or even her carnal desires. Women's secrets ranging from painkillers to hair strengtheners came from daily life and gradually developed into a part of the oral traditions of the world's women.

Ancient Egypt is where we begin to get our first consistent evidence about ancient cosmetic uses. There, cosmetic use was the norm, not the exception. The Egyptians developed a highly sophisticated system that is at the basis of many of our modern cosmetics. The Ebers Papyrus, an Egyptian medical text that is one of the world's oldest, offers recipes for everything from correcting a displaced uterus to curing baldness. Aside from the medical necessities common to humankind, the Egyptians' beauty secrets grew out of a twofold aim: protection from the fierce desert climate in which they lived and a religious need to preserve the dead from decay. The result was a beauty arsenal that would rival those of today's most dedicated supermodel.

A glance inside the cosmetic case of Thutu, wife of Ani, who lived in the thirteenth century B.C., reveals the extent to which Egyptians had developed the art of beauty. There were special slippers for her comfort during the application of her makeup. There were elbow cushions to be used as armrests while her servants made up her eyes, and a pumice stone, which was used to remove body hair as well as to smooth rough skin on elbows, knees, and feet. There are empty cosmetic pots of alabaster and semiprecious stones that would have been filled with unguents and facial creams. Some of these were Coan quince cream, used by great ladies to smooth their complexions, *psagdi,* a perfumed ointment, and *aegyptium,* a popular hand and face cream. Unfortunately, the ingredients of these and other Egyptian cosmetics have been lost in time.

Thutu, as any well-born Egyptian woman would be, was very careful about her eye makeup. It was, after all, not only an enhancement of her beauty; it also protected her eyes. Eye pencils were made of wood or ivory and used to apply the shadow powder that was worn in damp weather. During sunnier times, a colored liquid protected the eyes from the sun's glare and gave birth to the Egyptian look that Elizabeth Taylor would emulate millennia later. A bronze mixing dish enabled Thutu to create just the right color. She, like the great beauty Nefertiti, would ring the eyes with a green cosmetic of now-unknown composition, then outline them with galena, a dark gray lead ore that was drawn into winged lines at the outer corners of the eye. The Ebers Papyrus echoes Thutu's concern about her eyes, devoting much time to diseases of the eyes, including blindness, bleary eyes, and cataracts. A remedy for bloodshot eyes called for two clay vessels. One was to be filled with powdered fruit of the doum palm and the milk of a woman who had borne a son. The other was to be filled with cow's milk. The eyes were to be bathed with the doum palm fruit mixture each morning and then washed with the cow's milk four times daily for six days. Try asking for that at your beauty counter.

Eyes prepared, Thutu would have probably turned her attention to the rest of her face and body. Cheeks and lips would have been stained with a mixture of red ocher and oil. Her hands and fingernails would have been reddened with a henna mixture, and her nipples would have been gilded. Toilet complete, Thutu would have been ready to go out, perhaps carrying some small beads of bdellium resin in her bag as a solid perfume.

Thutu is but one of Egypt's many beauties. Each brought her own innovations to the growing world of beauty. Queen Ses, mother of King Teta, was the first recorded user of henna as a hair dye. She is also mentioned in the Ebers Papyrus as being one for whom a cure for baldness was devised (no connection, one hopes). In the minds of the Western world, Cleopatra is the symbol of Egyptian beauty. Her beauty secrets ranged from using bear grease (natural lanolin) to make her hair grow, to the lavish use of her personal scent: a mixture of sandalwood, winter's bark, orrisroot, patchouli, myrrh, woodrose, and olibanum. This she burned in braziers and kept in large bowls as a potpourri, like traditional women in today's Senegal and Mali, who use their own special *thiouraye* to personalize their linens and their homes.

The Hebrews, when they settled in the Holy Land, took with them Egyptian ideas of perfumery. However, these oils and unguents were for religious use only. The daughters of Israel were not to use them. Those, like Jezebel, who dressed in scarlet, decked themselves with ornaments of gold, and enlarged their eyes with paint were doomed. It's a small wonder, then, that when the Queen of Sheba appeared, she enchanted. Her lips "dropped as the honeycomb," and the smell of her garments was like the "smell of Lebanon." She brought with her all the spices, oils, unguents, and essences of the Eastern cultures as well as the woman-knowledge of their special secrets that captivated King Solomon. She brought a bit of the air of the exotic world.

Egyptians cared for their bodies. As the aesthetic was for a smooth body, all body hair was removed for comfort as well as hygiene. The Egyptians were also the first to codify the art of tattooing. They developed the art of puncturing the skin and inserting a permanent dye under it between 4000 and 2000 B.C.

All Egyptian women knew the importance of personal cleanliness and bathed several times daily, including before and after meals. Baths were accompanied by a scrub-down with fine sand and finished off by trips to unguent rooms, where the body was perfumed with aromatic oils. The Egyptians believed that the living body must be cared for in life so that it could be maintained in death. All the bathing, though, prompted the Greek historian Herodotus to comment that they "set cleanliness above seemliness."

Cleanliness has always been a hallmark of the beauty of the exotic world. In regions such as the Middle East, North Africa, Pakistan, and wherever Islam has spread, there are specific recommendations as to the frequency and method of bathing. Unguents and oils were devised to enhance the bathing experience. As early European explorers came to know more about Eastern ways, the dominion of the perfumes expanded to include the Western world.

The chemists and alchemists of the Arab world developed the process of distillation in the ninth and tenth centuries. Yakub al-Kindi left a work entitled *Kitah Kimiya' al'-Itr wa'l-Tas'idat* or *The Book of Perfume Chemistry and Distillation,* in which he discusses the distillation of attar of roses. A tenth-century Arab doctor, Avicenna, is also credited with being one of the first to distill floral scents. These Arab chemists turned the Middle East into a perfumed garden. Vast quantities of musk were mixed with the mortar of the mosque of Zobaide at Tarsus and the mosque of Kara Amed, and the buildings thrilled with a lushness of scent rarely equaled since. The fragrance in many of them lingers even today.

While musk was the scent that pervaded the buildings, the scent that captivated the people was rose. The prophet Mohammed is believed to have said, "When I was taken up to Heaven, some of my sweat fell on the earth and from it sprang the rose, and whoever would smell my scent, let him smell the rose." Indeed, some strands from his beard are enshrined at the mosque of Omar in Jerusalem, and they still retain the faint scent of rose.

The seclusion of the harem and its emphasis on the world of beauty led many Arab women into devising cosmetics and perfumes to enhance themselves. Their formidable beauty preparations and cosmetics included *hemsia,* an almond unguent used as a cleansing cream. *Hemsia* was also pressed into the navel to perfume it. Teeth were cleaned with *souek,* a tooth powder made from the bark of the walnut tree. This is still available in markets in North Africa and the Middle East, and is used as chew sticks as well. Body hair was removed with *termentia,* a paste that contained turpentine, or with a honey-and-lemon paste that is still in use today. Hair was also removed by twisting a string and rubbing it along the part to be depilated. *Schnouda,* a face cream scented with jasmine, was used for a fresh complexion, while benzoin and pastilles called *kourss* were used as breath fresheners and also occasionally burned to perfume living areas.

In India, cosmetics were widely used for seduction as well. Vatsyayana, author of the love manual the *Kama Sutra,* records a vast selection of cosmetics. Women were enjoined to be skilled in sixty-four extra arts of seduction, along with the knowledge imparted in the *Kama Sutra* itself. These arts included tattooing, coloring hair, nails, and bodies, and "applying perfumed ointments to the body." The *Kama Sutra* is so specific about the necessity for cosmetics as a part of a woman's sexual arsenal that recipes for particular cosmetics are included in the text. One relates the ingredients for the preparation of a mascaralike cosmetic with all the seriousness that would be accorded a magic potion.

Muslim bridegrooms in India were even required to present their brides-to-be with a *singardan* or toilet bag. The bag contained a *pandam,* or box for betel nut (a breath freshener), a bottle of attar of roses, and a casting bottle for sprinkling rose water on guests. Traditionally, there are also three cosmetics boxes: one for *kajal* or kohl, an eye cosmetic; one for *soorma,* an eye shadow; and one for the teeth-blackening powder that was used by married women. The *singardan* also held a comb, a mirror, brushes, and other cosmetic implements—in short, everything a woman might need to be beautiful.

While Egyptians used cosmetics for religious reasons and to protect themselves from the sun, many scholars believe that cosmetics strictly for adornment as we know them today may have originated in China over four thousand years ago. For many centuries, upper-class Chinese women considered putting on heavy makeup as natural as getting dressed in the morning. In Peking in the thirteenth century, upper-class women anointed their faces in the wintertime with a paste that was called "Buddha adornment." The paste remained on until the spring, when it was removed to reveal a complexion that was alleged to be as smooth and lustrous as jade. In the more southern regions near Hangzhou, women applied a coat of white powder called *meen-fung* to their faces, then added touches of carmine to the cheeks, lips, nostrils, and even the tongue. Eyebrows were usually tweezed and then redrawn with a pencil or charcoal and arched to resemble a willow leaf. A light dusting of rice powder was the finishing touch to set the makeup and soften the effect.

Chinese women recognized the need for skin care from an early date. They maintained their complexions by applying a mixture of tea oil and rice powder before retiring. The masque was removed in the morning before the makeup was applied. Makeup was so much a part of the lives of traditional upper-class Chinese women that it was *not* worn only when they were in mourning and, ironically, on their wedding days.

Japanese women, like their Chinese sisters, evolved an extensive beauty ritual that is still practiced by geisha today. Their system of beauty used many techniques that are only now being discovered by the West. Centuries ago, they developed methods of facial massage, a practice that only recently began to be investigated by Western cosmetologists. Japanese women also understood that feeding the inner woman developed the beauty of the outer woman and thought that eating kelp and seafood would contribute to the glossiness of their hair. Mineral baths were known and their benefits understood. Complex perfume ceremonies invited participants to guess certain scents and to associate them with seasons, works of literature, and the like. The arts of dressing and hairstyle were codified so that each change of color, outfit, or hairstyle signaled something to those cultivated enough to be in the know. The arts of traditional beauty particularly flourished at the courts and in Yoshirawa—the Ukiyo-e or Floating World, a famous pleasure section of Yedo, or Old Tokyo. This was the world of the geisha, with their beautiful, yet strictly defined, makeup and garments. During much of the nineteenth century, the section certainly must have been one of the beauty high spots of the Far East.

The cosmetic arts flourished in the New World, too. The diaries and codices of the priests and explorers who first visited the Americas indicate that the women were alluring. In the Caribbean region, clothing was minimal; body paint and feathers were used for adornment. *Roucou,* a red dye prepared from the *achiote* or annatto plant (*Bixa orellana*), was used to tint lips and body. It is thought to have kept the insects at bay as well. On the South American continent, the flourishing Native American civilizations had even more to teach Europeans.

During excavations of pre-Incan graves in Peru, a mummy of a young woman was discovered. The young woman was of the Moujik people who lived around 500 B.C. Her body was dressed in a lace gown, wrapped in yards of lace, and then covered with mummy cloth and cotton net. Her hair was cut into a bob, and she had plucked eyebrows, manicured and polished fingernails and toenails, as well as reddened cheeks and lips. In the same grave, the young woman's toilet case was discovered. In it she had a container for face powder and a powder puff of soft feathers, a tube filled with lip color (which had dried up) and a small silver implement for applying it, a container of a rougelike paint, and one holding a dark black pigment that was used for the eyebrows. The toilet case's contents were rounded out by a pair of tweezerlike tools, a bronze nail-paring knife, and a hardwood cuticle stick. Clearly, beauty was a priority in this hemisphere many years before Columbus got lost and happened across it.

The Aztec civilization's numerous bathing facilities startled the Spanish explorers. (In the late fifteenth and early sixteenth centuries, bathing was still far from common in Europe.) Aztec women were also meticulous about their appearance. They used a cosmetic called *axim* to enhance their complexions, burned a fragrant tree resin called copal to purify the air in their homes, conditioned their hair with jojoba oil, and used the avocado from peel to pit to beautify themselves.

In the north, Native Americans not only instructed settlers in survival skills, they also showed them how to use soap root as a mild shampoo, to roll the leaves of the *yerba santa* plant and chew them as a refreshing mouthwash, and to use chaparral (creosote) as a dandruff-treating hair tonic. Women learned to brew a tea of pennyroyal and dandelion to relieve menstrual cramps. The settlers learned more, much, much more, and many Native American practices went on to form a large part of the American natural-cosmetic arsenal.

Slavery, the largest forced migration of people in history, would unite three worlds—Native American, African, and European—and would result in the development of variations on the traditional cosmetics of each. The enslaved Africans, though, also retained many of the ways of their African homelands. Dutertre, a French colonial observer, recorded that some slaves attached their hair with strings.

> They only find themselves beautiful when they have 60 or so
> of those cotton cords which tie their hair, in bunches as thick
> as a little finger together. From afar, one would mistake their
> heads for those of a Medusa.

Dutertre was less than taken with the hairstyle. He might have liked it a bit more had he known that the slaves were simply following an old African custom of wrapping the hair to keep it in place and to make it grow. This style, which is still very popular in Benin and Togo, is returning to the United States. It is, in fact, a perfect way to give extremely damaged hair a rest and still look chic.

Dutertre recounts another slave habit: "Men and women alike rub the whole body with palm oil in order to appear blacker." It is debatable whether palm oil makes the skin appear blacker. What it does do is add sheen and vitality to complexions made dark and ashy from too much sun or too much cold. Palm oil is still used in this way in many parts of Africa. (In America, Vaseline and other store-bought emollients, from Crisco to Chanel's Cristalle body lotion, have taken over this use.) Palm oil is used indirectly as a skin enhancer in Brazil as well. There, the descendants of slaves who live in the northeastern section of the country call it *dende* and use it in cooking. Its culinary use is said to give the women of the Northeast their particular glowing complexions. In the West, though, palm oil in the diet has come under fire from some nutritionists, although its emollient qualities have been noted. It is an ingredient in many commercial soaps, where it functions as a skin softener. In fact, the original formula for Palmolive soap included both palm and olive oils—hence the soap's name.

For generations, African cosmetics rituals were kept intact in the New World by the slaves and their descendants. In many cases, they were aided by the sub-rosa retention of African religious rites, which maintained a close link with the plant world and the traditional herbal medicine of the mother country. Ritual baths were regularly prescribed by practitioners. There were baths for healing and for spiritual cleansing, as well as baths for love, for success in any endeavor, and for the myriad other occurrences that are a part of daily life.

Aside from the religious practitioners, there was always an older woman somewhere close by who knew which concoction to brew if a girl "got into trouble," or how to help milk return to dry breasts, or how to enhance one's attributes. Their methods worked and their fame spread. Gradually, the plantations' mistresses and their daughters began to look, not only to their European beauty cases, but also to their slaves for advice on cosmetics and special hints on how to adjust to the rigors of living in the tropics.

Descendants of these women are still active today. They are the *curanderas* of the Mercado San Juan in Mexico City; the *mambos* of Carrefour, Haiti; the *madrinas* of Matanzas, Cuba, and Loíza Aldea, Puerto Rico; the *maes de santo* of Salvador da Bahia, Brazil; and the root workers of South Carolina's Sea Islands, Louisiana's bayous, and the urban inner cities of the southern and northern metropolises of the hemisphere. Herbal wonder-women—they are the keepers of many of the beauty secrets and the pharmacology of the western half of the exotic world.

These women and their foremothers are a vital part of the history of the hemisphere, for they, who were more familiar with the climate and the flora and lived closer to the land, helped European women adjust to new lives in new lands. During the colonial period, many of the women who had been nursed by these women of color, and who had learned some of the arts of exotic beauty from them, returned to Europe and took some of their secrets with them. They fascinated and scandalized the European world. Under the French Directory, Madame Thérèse Tallien was one such woman. A Creole from Martinique, she was the beauty arbiter of her day and a scandalous one at that. She would luxuriate in baths of strawberries and raspberries and then be gently rubbed with sponges soaked in perfumed milk. Her contemporary, arguably the most famous white Creole woman of the late eighteenth and early nineteenth centuries, was Marie-Josèphe-Rose Tascher de la Pagerie of Trois-Îlets, Martinique. (The most famous Creole of color was certainly Marie Laveau, who by profession was a hairdresser.)

Marie-Josèphe-Rose Tascher would go on to become, first, Joséphine de Beauharnais, wife of a Parisian aristocrat executed during the French Revolution. But it was in her second husband that she met her true destiny, for he was Napoleon Bonaparte, and she would become the empress Joséphine. Not conforming to the pallor that was the accepted beauty canon of her day, she relaunched the fashion for rouge and in one year alone spent almost three thousand francs on the cosmetic, a staggering figure. Rouge, though, was far from Joséphine's only cosmetic passion. She was extremely fond of musk perfume, a throwback perhaps to the headier scents of the tropics of her birth. She used so much musk perfume that her rooms at Malmaison smelled of musk for years after her death. One story has it that Napoleon couldn't stand the fragrance and she doused her room in it as revenge after he divorced her. She also shared in the love of adornment that enhances the beauty of many women of the exotic world. Her clothing bills were legendary, and her love for Indian paisley shawls was the subject of more than one stern letter from her husband.

Joséphine Bonaparte and Thérèse Tallien were not exceptions. The languor and beauty of the Creole women were sung by poets and novelists of the period. Joséphine's distant cousin, school friend, and fellow Martiniquaise, Aimée du Buc de Riverny, after an amazing series of quirks of fate became the favorite of Sultan Selim III of Constantinople. In the nineteenth century, Baudelaire maintained a lifelong love for Jeanne Duval, a mulatto woman. He wrote of her beauty in such poems as "La Chevelure" and "Parfum Exotique" in his collection *Fleurs du Mal.* He praised her sensuality in passionate verse that announced more than anything else that the European fascination with exotic women of color was beginning to come out into the open.

The later years of the nineteenth century and the early years of the twentieth would bring the world of exotic women of color out of "darkness" for Europeans and Americans. Colonial explorations, followed by colonial expositions and world's fairs, would make places like Egypt, India, French West and Equatorial Africa, Macao, the Gold Coast, and Hong Kong more familiar, albeit exotic, destinations. The maidens and memsahibs who traveled to India on the "fishing" fleets (so called because of the single young women who journeyed out to visit relatives in hopes of finding husbands) were thrown into contact with another world. The travels and the expositions acquainted more than one European woman with non-European ideas of beauty and adornment. Queen Victoria may not have wanted to use kohl, but she loved cashmere shawls with their musky, heady patchouli scent. Ubangi lips may have been derided, but British heiress Nancy Cunard, with her arms encased from wrist to elbow in heavy African bracelets, symbolized the avant-garde of an age. There was even a British vogue for tattoos among upper-class women, and more than one flapper experimented with a bit of kohl around her eyes.

Cosmetics manufacturers, ever mindful of promotional possibilities, sensed a boom in the making, and soon products began emerging with names that catered to the new fascination with the world of exotic beauty. Phul Nana and Shem-el-nessim were two inexpensive scents launched on the awaiting public in the early twentieth century. At the other end of the fragrance spectrum, the great house of Guerlain created perfumes for the upper classes based on the same marketing concept. Mitsouko (1919) evoked the mysteries of Japan; Shalimar (1925) spoke of the eternal loves of the Indian subcontinent; and Liu (1929) called forth imperial China, as it was named for the Chinese slave girl of the opera *Turandot.* All promised delights based on names that invoked the pleasures of the forbidden seraglio and suggested a sensuality that had been heretofore taboo (the name of a 1931 fragrance, Tabu). Their heavy oriental scents were a far cry from the lavender water that was previously popular.

And then a little more than a century after it adored Joséphine Bonaparte, Europe fell under the spell of another Josephine, "La Baker." She and other less well known African American performing artists, such as Florence Mills and Bricktop, used traditional African American beauty methods and even invented some new ones. Josephine Baker was particularly fond of the beauty secrets of exotic women of color. She used kohl on her eyes, as did Theda Bara, the legendary vamp of the 1920s. La Baker tried the Islamic fashion for henna on her hands but abandoned it after it smeared some costumes, and even considered having her lips tattooed red to save time by not having to apply lipstick. She decided against tattooing when she learned that the process would be quite painful.

Europe began a love affair with exotic beauty as a result of the French colonial expositions: those of Marseilles in 1906 and 1922 and the style-defining mother of them all, the Exposition Coloniale Internationale of Paris in 1931. There, European women came face-to-face with their counterparts from the world of women of color. Women from French Indochina rubbed shoulders with those from French West Africa and French Equatorial Africa and those from the French West Indies. European women observed them all, and the Western world of beauty took note. Movies and photographs acquainted people with new destinations, and new looks and fashions were launched. The Great Depression, followed by World War II, brought a stop to much, but in the late 1940s and the 1950s a fascination with the beauty regimens of exotic women of color, both contemporary and historical, would grow again. Two versions of the story of Cleopatra, one by Vivien Leigh in the 1950s and another that launched the Elizabeth Taylor–Richard Burton love saga in the 1960s, transformed eye makeup. By the 1960s Elizabeth Taylor's Cleopatra look, a direct adaptation of the makeup technique shown in Egyptian tomb paintings, launched the vogue for dark black eyeliner with winged corners. Even a performer as mainstream as Lucille Ball made her use of a henna rinse a household joke.

In the late 1950s and the 1960s, African American models began to appear. Donyale Luna captivated France and the world. Cosmetics companies, scenting a change in the wind, began to research the beauty practices of women of color, looking for new product ideas.

The flower-child culture of the 1960s looked to the East for spiritual inspiration and found a whole new world of beauty. Kohls and *kajals* were used to decorate the eyes. Body painting, a throwback to the earliest forms of makeup, had a brief upsurge. Female body tattooing with small and then larger designs was yet another way of showing independence. Multiple ear piercings, perhaps a gift from the Toucouleur and the Fulani of West Africa, became a craze. From the Middle East, natural oils and essences were adopted to perfume the body, and the whole decade reeked of musk and patchouli oils—both the superexpensive essential oils and the mock—as a new generation of women found that these essences were longer-lasting than perfume and could be personalized in innovative ways. Incense, long a tradition in the East, the Near East, and other parts of the exotic world, was used to hide the smell of marijuana smoke and became traditional in many Western houses as well.

The Black Revolution of the sixties and seventies not only raised consciousness about civil rights, it also made some think of their origins, not to mention their roots. Cornrows and other hairstyles that only grandmothers could administer accompanied by a solid thwack of the back of the brush were worn with pride as the Afro segued into a renaissance of African and African-inspired hairstyles. Hair braiding, hair wrapping, and cornrowing were revived and later joined by box braiding and dreadlocks. Grandmothers, great-aunts, and mothers were being asked about traditional secrets. People began to use powdered brewer's yeast mixed with water as a facial masque. The egg-white facial masque, one that can be traced as far back as ancient Egypt, made a comeback as well. Mayonnaise came out of the refrigerator and became a hair conditioner, and the avocado found its way into a lot more than salads. Models of color strutted their stuff on catwalks and startled the world with their sleek look and their ability to wear clothes in new, innovative ways.

Increased ecological and health awareness in the 1970s produced a desire for natural products unadulterated with chemical additives. Concern for animal rights also made women aware of animal testing; many revised their cosmetics-buying habits, forcing companies to change their policies. As the women's movement increased knowledge about women all over the world, eyes were once again turned to women of color, and they responded with an outpouring of knowledge. *Herbal* became a watchword that was a must for many a cosmetic advertisement, and the race was on. Traditional beauty secrets from Native Americans gave us jojoba oil and yucca shampoos. Madeline Mono founded an empire on the kohl and *kajal* of Indian women. Companies released products that were direct adaptations of Moroccan kohl and *akkar* (a cheek stain). A multipurpose claylike substance called Indian

Earth was promoted as being able to work as everything from a body high-lighter to a nail stain. Henna had a rebirth, and colored hennas became a brief fad within the hair-care industry.

The 1980s brought us *botanicals* as a cosmetic watchword, as more and more Westerners recognized the cornucopia of cosmetic know-how represented by women of the exotic world. Tattooing was also brought back in fashion. No one but friends and lovers, masseuses and morticians know what designs adorn the Chanel-suited bodies of many a yuppie stockbroker and lawyer. Where only decades ago tattoo parlors were slightly seedy places frequented by thugs and drunken sailors, today even the famous are submitting to the designer's needle. As one tattoo-savvy sage put it, "In the sixties you got tattooed to be out. Now you get tattooed to be in." Many have gone beyond tattooing to piercing—and not simply ears or noses. Today, pierced navels and eyebrows are increasingly common.

Ann Roddick, owner of the Body Shop chain of cosmetics boutiques, declares in an advertisement on national television in the United States that majority-world notions of beauty take her breath away. Bennetton, an Italian knitwear company, builds its advertising look on the juxtaposition of star-tling young faces from Senegal, Vietnam, Togo, Mexico, and the like with their European counterparts. An American edition of *Elle* debuts, and faces of models like Beverly Peele, Naomi Campbell, and Julie Shimada challenge Western notions of beauty and let the world know that the beauty of women of color has come to the forefront again.

While many look to the world's women of color for beauty secrets, even more look to them for wardrobe ideas. With the increasing accessibility of air travel, ethnic dressing has reserved its place in virtually everyone's closet. Large stores have responded with folkloric boutiques, and smaller ones thrive on imported exotica alone. Caftans are common for formal wear; kimonos double as evening wear; Chinese quilted jackets are winter news. Ponchos, heavy Ecuadoran sweaters, and Mexican rebozos keep off autumn chills. De-signers from Poiret to Ralph Lauren have taken their cues from the women of the exotic world. With the rising price of gold, silver ethnic jewelry is the thing. The jewelry of the peoples of the southwestern United States has be-come so popular, in fact, that it is now priced out of the range of many. Antique ivory bracelets of the Nancy Cunard type are now considered by some to be verboten and by others to be representations of their African heritage. When they can be found, they are very collectible indeed. West African glass trade beads, Ethiopian Coptic crosses, silver bangles and belts from the Indian subcontinent, delicate silver filigree from Southeast Asia, gold earrings from the French Antilles, jade from China, and more appear on one and all.

Anyone who has flown back from Jamaica or St. Thomas in the dead of winter knows that Bo Derek's transformation from a 6 to a 10 marked more than one woman. The interiors of northward-bound planes simply click with the knocking together of hundreds of tiny beads that are affixed to the braided hair of most of the American, European, and Canadian women. On the north coast of Jamaica, hair braiding is so much in style that there are government-established braiding centers where tourists can go to have a braid or two put in, or their entire heads done.

The perfumers have also caught on, and the musk oil of the sixties and seventies seems tame compared with fragrances known as Kif and Opium and Poison. Orientalism has crept back in with Casmir by Chopard, a 1990s fragrance that boasts of its use of the lotus, "flower of the east, mirror of the soul." The 1960s cosmetic Indian Earth has been reissued, complete with new advertising copy stressing that it is a natural product. Again, we're look-ing to the world of exotic women.

Coming from cultural attitudes, religious rituals, and climatic necessi-ties as well as external practices, the traditional beauty of women of color re-lies on centuries of beauty formulas and suggestions that inform women about everything from eye makeup to menopause, from inner peace to outer garments. These "secrets" have survived into the final decade of the twenti-eth century despite displacement, modernization, slavery, denigration, and the cultural steamroller known as progress. Now as the second millennium of the Christian era winds to a close, they are once again being examined and attempted and revered for the culturally and personally self-affirming wis-dom that they embody.

In this book we'll take a look at beauty rituals evolved over the ages by exotic women of color. We'll follow in the footsteps of Nefertiti, Cleopatra, Murasaki, Josephine Baker, and millions of other women in harems and huts, kitchens and courtyards, mansions and shanties throughout the exotic world. We'll look at their world of beauty and at them from inside to outside.

This book, though, is not just a history of the traditional beauty habits of women of color. It is also the testimony of a personal journey, a journey spanning more than forty years and five continents. This life's journey has gone from housing projects to palaces, temples to textbooks, on a quest for friendship with the women of the world. With their friendship came sister-hood, and with sisterhood came secrets shared.

My ongoing communion with my "sisters" around the world began over forty years ago on the day that my parents enrolled me in the United Nations International School. As the first student not connected with the United Nations, I grew up with those from other lands. I had girlfriends from India, Poland, England, Venezuela, Pakistan, Jamaica, Saudi Arabia, and other countries before I had close girlfriends in my own culture. Their countries became familiar to me even though I'd never visited them.

There was Shika's house, with its marvelous scent of turmeric mixed with sandalwood, where I first heard sitar music decades before George Harrison and others made Ravi Shankar a household word. I remember Shika's training in *bharata natya* and how the first time I saw her dance, I cried because my girlfriend had been transformed into a whirling goddess. I remember Vasu's house, with other smells of the subcontinent, and how her mother groomed her long silky braid with a special hair scrub and a coconut oil rinse. Shoba explained the meaning of the traditional Indian *tilak* or caste mark and showed me how to wrap a sari. I learned of other cultures from other friends. Sitting in their kitchens after school, I played and listened and soaked up things that would come back to me in a wave of familiarity years later as I began to travel the world. So many of the secrets of the world of women of color were learned in those childhood conversations.

When we all dispersed after idyllic childhoods in which world peace was a reality, not a dream, I went to the High School of Performing Arts in New York. There my favorite class was makeup. In it I learned about my own face, doing special geisha and Kabuki makeups and applying lines and shadows at age fifteen to attempt to see what I would look like at age fifty. (Now that I'm almost there, I know.) I remember slaving away at it one day when Vinette Carroll, the actress, whirled into the room like an avenging angel and loudly informed one and all that there was no need to teach African American students to studiously apply makeup base. "They already have the most fabulous base in the world!" she boomed out in her basso profundo. The words were affirming and would mark me for life, changing my thoughts about mainstream makeup, with its lack of cultural diversity. I would search out items from other cultures, and rice powder, *kumkum,* gold powders, kohl, and *kajal* would enter my makeup box and remain there.

As a college student in France, I would first come across the French-speaking world of women of color, along with different attitudes toward the beauty of the women of that world. I would see striking Senegalese matrons and svelte Creole women who accepted their beauty with fewer hangups than we seemed to have in the States. I would learn acceptance of myself and my cultural heritage from them.

The seventies marked my beginnings as a journalist and the start of my travels in the world of women of color. The decade began with trips to Haiti and Jamaica, and a West African odyssey that was designed to provide research for a doctoral dissertation but that provided knowledge about much more. Later in the seventies, I made excursions to most of the Caribbean, parts of West, East, and North Africa, Taiwan, Singapore, and Hong Kong, and the decade culminated in the miraculous discovery of Brazil.

Madras-clad market women in Fort-de-France, Martinique, revealed beauty hints involving cinnamon and vetiver. Newly made friends in Dakar and Cotonou showed hennaed hands, tattooed gums, and protective scars. A sophisticated Hong Kong beauty gave many hints, and when she ran out of them, she called her mother for more.

As a travel editor for *Essence* magazine in the late 1970s and early 1980s and then as a contributing editor to *Travel Weekly* in the mid-1980s, I crisscrossed the world, adding countries to my map, friends to my correspondence list, and beauty secrets to my knowledge. I walked through the bush in St. Croix one December with Leona Watson, a traditional herbalist who showed me the plants, picking small quantities of each so that I could take a luck-bringing bath for the new year. I watched wedding ceremonies in Jaipur and Delhi and even tasted betel nut, risking blackening my teeth. I journeyed to Haiti numerous times and spoke with many women there, spent many weeks and one hurricane in Jamaica, and took my first *hammam* in Morocco. I discovered the Afro-Brazilian religion of Candomblé in Salvador da Bahia, Brazil, and met the late Mae Menininha de Gantois, the woman known by many as the pope of Candomblé. I discovered Nonya culture and sarong *kebayas* in Singapore and invested heavily in Kanchipuram saris and silver belts in India, rode pillion on a motorbike from Rabat to Salé in Morocco to find a perfumer selling true essence of amber and musk, haunted antique shops and jewelry stores, beauty parlors, spas, and women's kitchens from Fès to Fort-de-France, Bahia to Brooklyn, Paris to Port-au-Prince, and Dakar to Delhi, with stops in Mombasa, Mexico City, Marrakech, and Miami.

In each place I made a friend, a girlfriend. In Agadir, Khadijah took me to the *hammam* after accompanying me to the market to buy what I needed. In Dakar, Theodora showed me where to get my hair braided and Nicole introduced me to her jeweler and her tailor. In Jamaica, Maria introduced me to her hairdresser and also to her mother. Aimee gave me protective tattoos in Ouidah, Benin, while her younger sister took me to the market to buy Nigerian cloth. In Bahia, Mae Tata, Kutu, Zurika, Celina, Tieta, and Sinha (who looks enough like me to be my blood sister) still guide me. I cannot return without remembering Mae Caetana, Mae Marinha, and beloved Vovo, who have since gone on to become ancestors. All of them took me in, instructed me, and initiated me into the ways of Candomblé. At each stop in my personal odyssey, I spoke with women using English, French, Spanish, and Portuguese, and when that failed, I turned to the international language of hand jive and a big smile. I learned that exotic beauty begins on the inside with a caring approach to life. Indeed, this is true of all beauty. I learned over the years that women around the world are as fascinated with the beauty hints of traditional women of color as I am.

The traditional beauty secrets of the exotic world are myriad. The ingredients are all natural. (The guide to mail-order sources in the back of the book will tell you where you can order items that may be hard to find where you live.) The processes are simple, and I have made a point to select recipes that can be easily followed. Most of them can be done alone. For some, though, you'll need a friend, but communion between women is very much a part of the beauty practices of the exotic world. You need no extra equipment to make these items. Everything can be done with things you already have in your kitchen or bathroom. The recipes are easy and they're fun. What's more, they come from the source, the place where it all started.

There are, alas, always a few caveats to remember. Your body and your body chemistry are uniquely your own. For that reason, a beauty recipe that has been used for centuries by women all over the world may not work for you. All recipes have been tested by me, but because your body chemistry is yours alone, test, test, TEST!

Before you use a recipe, dab a sample on a hidden spot about one inch square and leave it overnight. If there's no reaction, you're safe. If you get a rash, irritation, or other reaction, heed the warning. If you cannot eat tomatoes or avocados or use an ingredient mentioned in the recipes, don't use any of the recipes that call for that ingredient. I am allergic to spring grass and autumn ragweed and many things in between, and I almost did myself in once giving in to a friend's insistence that I try some of her miraculous bee pollen. I should have remembered, I'm allergic to pollen. THINK! We all have to be careful, but we can also enjoy the delights of exotic beauty. You'll find that not only do the recipes work toward a more beautiful you, many are also fun to make and have the extra benefit of being fresh each time they're used. After all, they haven't been around for centuries for no reason.

My friends, or their mothers and grandmothers, do not usually trouble themselves with teaspoons and tablespoons. They usually take a pinch of this and a handful of that and a few buds of the other. For purposes of simplification, though, and to make matters easier, I have used the traditional measures of teaspoons, tablespoons, and cups. When discussing essential oils, I have used drops. The recipes are good for one application unless otherwise stated.

These recipes come from women who experiment with them constantly; you should, too. Don't be afraid to change them; they are simply guides, not carved in stone. If you like the scent of lavender, add it to a bath oil or shampoo. If you hate patchouli, leave it out. Experiment. Many of these secrets have been around for centuries and they are as fluid as life itself. Remember also that all beauty products take time to act, including natural beauty products. There are no shortcuts, simply patience, consistent application, and common sense. You're only going to highlight the you that's already there.

Finally, don't forget the inner you that is the matrix of all beauty. Chapter 2 provides you with some ways to center yourself and offers words of advice and inspirational thoughts from international sources to tell you about being a woman and help you find the glow of inner peace that's recognized as true beauty in all the world's cultures. That's one of the most profound secrets: you are on the outside what you are on the inside. Make yourself the best possible person you can be and work to make it show. Start there, then go on to share my journey through the beauty world of exotic women of color.

Chapter 2

The Life Stages of Beauty

Child, Maiden, Lover, Mother, Crone

Love yourself;
Get outside yourself and take action.
Focus on the solution;
Be at Peace.   SIOUX TEACHING

Teaching should come from within instead of without.
HOPI SAYING

When you lose the rhythm of the drumbeat of God
You are lost from the peace and the rhythm of life.
CHEYENNE MAXIM

MY BRAZILIAN GODMOTHER is a spare woman with tiny bird bones, large all-seeing eyes that are deep pools of wisdom, and a face that can light up the world. A religious woman, she is the mistress and spiritual leader of one of the oldest houses of the Afro-Brazilian religion Candomblé in the town of Salvador da Bahia de Todos os Santos (better known as Bahia), Brazil. During my visits and stays in her religious house, she presides over ceremonials with a twist of her head, a slight raise of an eyebrow, or an imperious queenly gesture. In more informal moments, she is a quiet presence walking slowly and deliberately through the hallways of the main building, combing and recombing her hair.

Somehow the hair combing is particularly fitting, as her tutelary *oriṣa* is Oṣun, the Yoruba goddess of physical beauty. My godmother is not beautiful in the conventional manner, but when she sits on her carved mahogany throne attired in the traditional garments of her stature as supreme priestess and surrounded by the votaries of her religious house, she grows tall and impressive. Her openwork eyelet blouse, brightly colored flounced skirt, multiple heavily starched white petticoats, ropes of twinkling beads, shawl of handwoven Nigerian fabric, and head tie of a frothy white turban transform her into the queen of the world. Her spirituality and inner peace radiate from her all-seeing eyes, and she becomes a beacon of woman power beckoning all who see her to come and pay homage.

I am fortunate in my life to know many walking goddesses like my Brazilian godmother. You will meet some of them in the pages of this book. We all know goddesses who walk among us: our elders, our friends, our mothers, our sheroes. Most of us, though, do not know the goddess within, even though within each of us lives a goddess to be celebrated and saluted as much as any Aphrodite or Oṣun. Learn to identify your own goddess.

GODDESS IDENTIFICATION EXERCISE

Find a solitary spot in your house where you can be yourself and then find a full-length mirror and drag it there. Give yourself some quiet time, then take off all your clothes. Go ahead, don't be shy. I know it's difficult at first and seems funny, but do it for yourself. Now stand in front of the mirror and smile. Forget your blemishes and your "baby" fat and your love handles, pigeon toes, whatever you may have difficulty accepting. Smile, SMILE. . . . Do you see the goddess in you? Look harder; she's there.

She's the little girl you once were: serious or mischievous, solemn or sprightly. She's the adolescent you became, with all her secrets, her insecurities, and her delights in discovering her womanhood. She's the lover you are: tender, sensitive, sexy, vulnerable, and sensuous. She's the mother you are: loving, caring, nurturing, sustaining, and protective. She's the old woman you will become: wise, capable, commanding, majestic, and impressive.

Your inner goddess may be child, maiden, lover, mother, or crone in direct opposition to your actual chronological age. We've all seen young women who speak with the wisdom of years and older women who retain the inquisitiveness and joy of discovery of youth. It is the juxtaposition of interior goddess and individual that makes us unique.

Find your goddess. Look at her, love her, nurture her. Learn to see her smiling out from behind your eyes. Keep looking until you do. She's there—you just have to learn to take the time to see her and to salute her. Do it daily or weekly until you are comfortable with each other.

Child, Maiden, Lover, Mother, Crone—the goddess is a symbol of the potency of woman power, the awesome task of continuing and maintaining the life of the species. Women bring all humankind into the world. We carry our own unborn children under our hearts, then pass them along into the world. Those of us who are not birth mothers receive the children of others, nurture and care for them as though they were our own, and celebrate and rejoice with the waiting family. At the other end of time's spectrum, we take all humankind out, soothing grieving friends and family with nurturing hands, mourning, washing bodies, burying kinfolk and strangers alike. Whatever the culture, women are traditional fonts of nurturing and caring and the matrix of humanity. (If you don't believe me, think about the etymology of the word *matrix.*)

The art of being a woman has been transmitted from older women to younger ones since time began. It is the way that the young begin to see their inner goddesses. When young African girls become women, an integral part of the rite of passage is an intensive training period during which they are instructed in how to be women. Among Native American peoples, young women have elaborate coming-of-age ceremonies during which they learn about womanly virtues and women's secrets. The veil of purdah societies in India and the women's seclusion in many Muslim countries ironically allow transmission of womanly secrets from one generation to another, as do many family systems throughout the exotic world.

Woman-wisdom is transmitted orally throughout the cultures of the exotic world from the mouth of the elder to the ear of the younger, but sisters, cousins, aunts, godmothers, and just plain good friends frequently add their say. These words of wisdom are sustaining. They are what keep us going from the first time that a grandmother cries out, "Go on, baby girl," to the time that an aunt whispers, "Don't worry, honey, your mama did the same thing," to the painful times that a mother lifts a silent eyebrow and without uttering a word suggests that "a young lady never does that." They are some of the thoughts, words, and phrases that have nurtured the world's women.

The proverbs and admonitions of our upbringing are reflected in our daily lives. You will find some that sustain me as well as the nurturing thoughts of many cultures in these pages. Some of them may seem outdated or hopelessly tradition-bound. Others, though, may be refreshing—new thoughts for new times. Still others are amusing, designed to provide a smile when one is needed. Read them, consider them, look to them for comfort and even amusement. Don't ignore them, though; they're here to nurture your inner goddess. For as all women of the exotic world know, it is the inner essence that creates the outer woman. All the beauty secrets in the world are of no use if the inner woman is in turmoil. Feed your inner self on this spiritual food; savor it in the innermost recesses of your being. Drink deeply at the font of wisdom that springs from the goddesses who have walked among us on this earth. The cool, limpid spring of their wisdom will enhance not only your body, but your soul. And your soul is the true seat of your beauty.

DIVINE INSPIRATION

Exotic women bear the religious cultures of their people. Whether they worship the gods and goddesses of their foremothers or cling to the newer religions brought by colonial expansion, they have very special feelings about the sacredness of each and every day. They find beauty and meaning even in what seem to be the most mundane aspects of daily life. No item is too small to be considered.

Take time out each day to salute and admire the miracle of creation. No matter to whom or what you attribute them, contemplate the mysteries of a rose or a sunflower. Ponder the immensity of the ocean or the complexity of a butterfly. Learn the true meaning of the word *wonder.*

While I was staying in a Candomblé *terreiro* in Bahia, Brazil, I was struck by the daily devotion of the votaries of the Yoruba *oriṣa.* Each day began with a salute with prostrate body to the *oriṣa* of creation, Oxala, followed by a walk through the sacred precincts paying homage to the various sacred spots within the *terreiro.* I needed no alarm clock while there, for at 5:00 A.M. sharp the sibilant shuffling of slippers on the packed earth floor as they made their way signaled that the day had begun.

In India, many women begin each day with *pujas* or prayers, offering a garland of flowers or some food to their tutelary gods. Prayers may be formalized and prescribed at certain times throughout the day as they are in the Muslim world, or they may be gestures or thoughts that are as simple as burning a joss stick in the temple on the way to market or writing a thought or wish on a piece of paper and placing it in a sacred spot. The spiritual sustenance and wonder that come from the constant admiration of the miracle of creation give the woman of the exotic world an inner peace that is her sustaining lifeline.

In India, millions of people begin each day with a salute to the sun. They meditate on the radiance of the divine presence as expressed in the sun and ask that the fiery orb inspire and illumine not only their day but also their minds. Throughout the Muslim world, the muezzin's call, "Allah is great!" signals time for prayer at five prescribed times each day. The lunar calendar regulates the feast days and special observations of the Asian world, while in Haiti, Brazil, Cuba, Trinidad, Benin, Puerto Rico, Nigeria, and the United States, the sound of drumming invites people to celebrate the gods of the motherland. The cycle of observations may vary, the names of the divinities saluted may change, the pronunciation of the songs may alter, but the fervor and faith with which they are saluted is constant.

Some people are more comfortable with organized times of spiritual meditation and a calendar of observation. Others require more flexibility, and still others blend both into their own personal gospel, modifying it to grow as their needs require.

Find your own system. Learn what puts you most in touch with the universe. I found, only recently, that long slow walks along the beach or in the woods in my summer neighborhood on Martha's Vineyard allow me to talk to nature and feel at one with the world. In my urban environment, I've created a quiet place in my home where I can go. Try it yourself. Discipline yourself. So many of us have schedules that leave hardly one second that can be allotted to anything more. But take time; allow fifteen or twenty minutes a day. There's always time for your spiritual growth. My mother meditates in the bathtub after she's through washing. Try for the first thing in the morning or the last in the evening. Turn off the radio, the television, and your brain. Banish thoughts of unpaid bills and wars. Forget about family squabbles, friends' problems, and other cares and concerns. These minutes are for you to get in touch with yourself and your personal connections to the universe.

RELAXATION AND MEDITATION EXERCISE

Whatever your religious beliefs, this simple exercise will allow you to relax and give your inner self time to replenish.

Find a comfortable position on the floor or bed or even sitting in a favorite chair. Relax and close your eyes. Focus your mind on something you like, something that makes you smile. Think of a smooth beach stone, the sound of the waves in a conch shell, the rustle of the wind through leafy branches, the smell of a piñon fire, the feel of a velvet pillow or the rough fur of your first teddy bear, whatever you adore. These need not be present; you simply have to focus on them in your mind. When you've focused on your pleasant thought, then focus inward on giving yourself peace. Relax, slow down your breathing, calm yourself, replenish your essence, and gather strength. Begin by relaxing your toes and feet, pass onward to your legs, and then upward to your torso and upper body. Empty your mind of everyday cares and mentally focus on what makes you smile. When you find your focus fading, slowly begin to allow the world to return to you: open your eyes and look around, reacquaint yourself with your surroundings, and return to life and to work.

Whatever method you use to relax and get in touch with yourself, you'll find that this quiet time will sustain you and that you will look forward to it and grow with it. In fact, this quiet time may become indispensable to your inner well-being.

THE ASPECTS OF WOMAN

Throughout the world, women are culture bearers. They transmit the history and the tradition of the people down through the generations. They are the heart of the home and the matrix of the family. The Vedas, a holy book of the Hindus, state simply and accurately that "the wife is the home." Indeed, hers is the pivotal position of culture bearer and home maker (not in the abused, one-word, 1950s sense of that term, please). Over the span of their lives, whether as princesses or beggars, doctors or ditchdiggers, homemakers or heartbreakers, women learn and grow.

Child, Maiden, Lover, Mother, Crone. The archetypical goddesses reappear within our own personal life spans. The Child greets the world with inquisitiveness, certainty, and all the clear-eyed freshness of youth. The Maiden senses the changes in herself and in the world around her and begins to assume her role in the circle of women. The Lover combines the knowledge of sensuality and coquetry with the quiet, wistful knowledge of loves lost. The Mother nurtures and empowers all humankind and gazes on

prayer, dancing, and instruction. A female attendant is chosen to serve as godmother to the young woman. It is her task to dress, feed, care for, and teach her charge the ways of women. During these ceremonies, the young woman is identified with White Painted Woman, who is also called Changing Woman and White Shell Woman. It is this identification that is symbolized by the dress the young woman wears, which is made of yellow buckskin and sewn by her mother, grandmother, or other female relative. At times during the four-day ceremony, the young woman is painted with white chalk. During this period, she is thought to possess special healing powers and helps those who come to her.

In our Western society, these rites of passage have mainly disappeared. Indeed, this disappearance is but one signal of the breaking of the circle of transmission of woman-knowledge: the power and beauty both inner and outer that reside in the simple fact of being a woman. The circle can be reestablished when we rediscover the coming-of-age rituals of our foremothers or create new ones for our times.

While we now come from many different religious backgrounds and tribes, we share in the need to mark special anniversaries in our lives. Invite a young woman that you know well to have a special ceremony celebrating her first menstruation. Be creative and do something special. Consider the following rite of passage.

RITE OF PASSAGE FOR A YOUNG WOMAN

After you find that your daughter, sister, niece, or young girlfriend has had her first period, invite her to your home for a woman's meal. It may be a lunch, a dinner, or even a fancy afternoon tea. Invite several of your closest women friends to join you on this special day, and ask them to bring woman-gifts for the young woman: soothing herbal baths, empowering books, fancy undies, perfumes or perfumed oils, and the like. Ask each of your friends to be prepared to tell a brief story of her experiences with her own period or to read a passage from a book or poem that talks of woman's cyclical relationship to the universe. (Some passages from Maya Angelou's *I Know Why the Caged Bird Sings* or Ntozake Shange's *Sassafrass, Cypress, and Indigo* are particularly appropriate.) Spend the afternoon with the young woman laughing, talking, joking, and welcoming her joyously into the world of women.

Child, Maiden, Lover, Mother, Crone, the aspects of womankind are an ever-moving circle. Nurture it.

Lover

Nothing brings out a woman's natural beauty like love. Yes, sure, it's a cliché, but it is also a truism. All the beauty secrets in the world take a backseat to the glow that love can produce. There are many types of love, including sexual love and nurturing mother love (we'll deal with this in the next aspect), and the most important love of all, self-love.

Throughout the centuries and the cultures of the world, love has been celebrated and revered. Works like the Indian *Kama Sutra* (Scripture of love) of Vatsyayana and the *Amanga Ranga* have offered wisdom to generations of lovers, suggesting that they avail themselves of all their senses in the art of making love. In the fourteenth century, Sheikh Nefazawi discussed the use of perfumes and oils in enhancing the pleasure of lovemaking. Even a work as seemingly staid as the Christian Bible contributes some suggestions: consider Proverbs 7 or the erotic verses of King Solomon in the Song of Songs. Women of color have offered myriad hints for the lover, from seductive baths and massage oils to special hints for keeping a lover. For some of these, see chapters 6 and 7. The world of women also provides some rueful advice about how to deal with lost lovers.

It seems as though whenever two or more women are together for longer than two hours, some time is spent talking about men, what they do, and, more often than not, what they don't do. If love can give a glow like nothing else, it can also take it away. A Congolese proverb says, "To love someone who doesn't love you is like shaking a tree to make the dewdrops fall."

The African American South, the culture that spawned the blues, a music that has transformed love lost into a high art form, offers many lover's laments in the form of song. They make perfect listening for those days when things are just not going right. Listening to the blues, though, does not mean singing the blues about lost love.

Over the years, women have come up with several suggestions for solving the problem of lost loves. My friend Martha, who is nothing if not outspoken, reminded me of this one.

THREE THINGS NOT TO DO FOR A MAN

Don't *buy him a mattress. . . .*
He'll only use it with his other girlfriend!

Don't *send him to school. . . .*
He'll just get uppity and put you down!

Above all, don't buy him shoes. . . .
He'll just walk out of your life!

Some folks still don't give shoes because of this, and if they do, the recipient must pay a token two cents so that he won't walk out.

Southern sayings aside, love is vital. It is as necessary as oxygen. Loving and being loved do more for creating inner peace and outer beauty than all the cosmetics in the world. There are simply two things to remember. In the fourth century, Saint Augustine said, "There is no greater invitation to love than loving first." He was right. Only a few weeks ago my mother said, "Love is the key to beauty, indeed the key to life, but before you can love anyone or anything, you must learn to love yourself in all of your intricate splendor." That says it all.

LOVER'S REMINDERS

On small blank white index cards, write down the ten things that you like best about yourself and the ten things that you consider to be most lovable about yourself. Then scatter the cards in places where you will find them as you go about your day's business: in the corner of the bathroom mirror, on the dashboard of your car, near the telephone, by the alarm clock. Each time you see one, read it softly to yourself, smile, and know that you are lovable and that you are loved.

Child, Maiden, Lover, Mother, Crone, the aspects of womankind are a kaleidoscope of possibilities. Grow with them.

Mother

Mother love—there's nothing like it. Whether it is the affection of a physical mother or a spiritual mentor, those who have basked in its warmth can testify to its almost tangible strength. Mother and child form a unit so powerful that it has become totemic in almost all the world's religions. In most traditional societies, children nurse at their mothers' breasts, thereby developing bonds that last a lifetime. In West Africa, one of the first things many foreigners notice is that there are few events that babies do not attend. They travel to market comfortably strapped to their mothers' backs, heads lolling in a way that drives many Westerners to distraction. There, they sleep under market stalls while their mothers ply their wares. Young girls who are barely able to toddle follow their mothers around and imitate them in their daily activities. They strap their younger siblings to their backs and play at sweeping in the courtyard. They also imitate their mothers in their beauty rituals, braiding each other's hair, tying and retying each other's *pagnes,* and pretending that they are grown up. Their mothers help them, assigning them tasks that grow with their abilities. In this way, mothers guide their daughters, making sure that they are versed not only in secular ways, but in the ways of the inner woman as well. Think of your own youth, remember playing dress-up, and the ways that you learned how to be a woman from the advice that your mother gave you.

Mwana Kupona, the wife of a well-known Swahili sheikh, lived from 1810 to 1860 on Siu, a small island off Lamu, another island off the coast of Kenya. Two years before dying, she wrote an epic poem in Swahili to her daughter, Mwana Hashima Binti Sheikh, who was one of her delights. In it she gives her the mother-to-daughter advice that she felt she would not be able to offer in times of need. The *Utendi Wa Mwana Kupona* is a classic Swahili poem or *tendi,* but the message is a universal one that could have been repeated by generations of mothers to their daughters. In the poem, Mwana Kupona speaks to her daughter of how to live and how to behave. She tells her how to dress and adorn herself, offering her an amulet and a necklace of pearls and red coral to wear. She enjoins her daughter to hold fast to her faith and to follow the path of her religion. She entreats her to have a discreet tongue, to be truthful, and to avoid foolish people, "who do not know how to control themselves." In keeping with the time in which she wrote, Mwana Kupona tells her daughter to cater to her husband and be an asset to him.

Moreover, she advises her on matters of beauty, suggesting that she perfume herself with rose water and "dalia" powder and spread garlands of jasmine blossoms on the bed. She reminds her to always keep her fingernails hennaed and her eyes made up. "Do adorn yourself with finery that you remain like a bride," she begs. She was neither the first nor the last mother to urge her daughter on to higher concepts of beauty.

MOTHER'S MESSAGES

Whether we are birth mothers or not, most women have children. Our children, if they have not passed from our own loins, are our godchildren or the children that we teach in school, those of friends or of a religious community, those that we pass daily in our neighborhood or apartment buildings, or simply those we see as we go about our daily tasks. Think of a young woman in this group and compose a message for her. Work on it, revising it and reworking it as though you were Mwana Kupona writing for her daughter. How would you suggest that the young woman behave? What should she do to be happy in love? How should she comport herself in public? How should she dress and adorn herself?

As you write this message, you are clarifying and fine-tuning for another generation the information that you received from your mother and from your life. You are also making statements about what you think is of value in your own code of behavior. If you have a daughter or know a young woman who is coming of age, write it up or have it written out and decorated by a calligrapher and present it to her. If there's no young woman in your life, hold on to it; there will be one someday.

Child, Maiden, Lover, Mother, Crone, the nurturing strength of woman-wisdom is empowering. Learn from it.

Crone

Wise and withered, dewlapped and diminutive, rotund and jolly, the gray-haired matriarchs of the world have long inspired awe with their wisdom and their presence. It is not without reason that most of the world's peoples think of the very earth on which we live as a primordial mother. These living ancestors are the wisdom of the earth that walks among us.

My grandmothers taught me more than I realized. Each day, I am surprised by the depth of what I learned unconsciously while I traveled in their shadows. They did it subtly, with a word, a proverb, or a look. My maternal grandmother, Grandma Jones, could put a hurtin' on some food. She had to. As a minister's wife, she had to feed not only her brood of twelve children but all those church sisters, traveling guest ministers, and anybody in the religious community in need as well—this at the height of the Depression (although, in truth, it was always a Depression for most people of color in the early part of the century in this country). She did it all and she did it well, baking industrial quantities of bread and seeing to it that everyone had enough, and keeping table conversation going with her witty and invariably sarcastic humor. When she had raised her own family, she decided to take up a career and went to beauty school to become a hairdresser. She worked at this until the travel bug bit and she worked at seeing as much of the world as possible. She was an avid clubwoman, finding ample scope for her impressive managerial skills in her handling of the Tents, the Eastern Star, the Moses Society, and more that I still don't know about. She kept in constant touch with her children and grandchildren and hosted a lengthy tableful of us all at holidays. She lived her life to the fullest. And when she'd done all she wanted to do and seen all she wanted to see, she died. In my family, we jokingly refer to a family tendency on the part of most Jones women suddenly to turn into whirling dervishes of activity upon reaching age forty. One aunt passed the mark and went back to school, completing a high school diploma, a college degree, and work on a doctorate in Asian studies that included mastering Sanskrit. My mother became a master jeweler specializing in miniature granulated pieces of cloisonnéd enamel after the age of sixty.

My paternal grandmother, Grandma Harris, was more conventional, but she found magic in everyday things. She could transform a blade of grass into a duck honk and skip stones with the best of them. She made her own lye soap and knew how to cornrow before it became fashionable. She also wrapped hair in a way that I only recently discovered harked back to our ancestors in western Africa. She too was a clubwoman, but more than that, she was mother to an entire neighborhood. One and all called her Mother Harris.

As with much of the richness of traditional life, I didn't realize how much it contributed to my own life until it was gone. It was only many years later that I saw that my Grandma Jones had prepared me for a future in which I could walk with princes and paupers alike with the same ease, one in which I could set an elegant table and carry on a witty conversation, all the while presenting a main dish that consisted of "doctored up" leftovers served so beautifully that no one would even suspect. My grandmother Harris was my link to the past. I realized that one day sitting in the Daniel Sorano Theatre in Dakar, Senegal. I heard a voice and it was my grandmother singing. It was as though she, who had been long dead, reached down out of the clouds and touched me with her hands. The timbre, the tone, the keening wail of the unknown Wolof singer captured the quintessence of the wordless songs that Grandma Harris hummed and half sang to herself as she went about her daily tasks. One grandmother had shown me the road to the future; the other had allowed me to look back into my past. Both had taught me about my own beauty and how to survive and keep it intact.

It was because of them that I am able even today to sit at the feet of wise old women around the world and listen and learn. Their wisdom is not always forthcoming, and they must take your measure before they speak. They look at you through rheumy eyes and gaze into your soul, determine whether you are sensitive to their knowledge or simply curious, read your heart and make their decisions. But if you are quiet, as I have learned to be, and if you sit spongelike, listening patiently and not interrupting with questions, all answers are forthcoming. The wisdom of the centuries is there in the words of these living goddesses, these walking history books, these women who are the repositories of the world's cultures and the world's traditional knowledge. An African sage has said that when an old person dies, it is as though a library has burned. The knowledge is irretrievable, whether it is knowledge of how to tie a turban in three swift movements, or how to heal a wound with a spiderweb, or how to paint hennaed designs on your hands that will signal your interest to a beau. Learn from them and keep the wisdom alive. Pass it on.

WISDOM QUEST

Find several older women, in your own lineage if possible, and invite them to a meal that you have prepared just for them. It may be a luncheon or simply a tea. Provide them with transportation if it's necessary and make sure that they know that this time is just for them. Prepare the room for their comfort and food that they will enjoy. Then after serving them, sit back and allow them to talk of their good times and their bad times, their beaux and their heartbreaks—in short, their lives. Let them ramble, digress, and reminisce as they journey back in time to when they were young. When they are comfortable, if you wish, you may gently ask a question or two about their beauty regimens, or about the way they prepared themselves for going out, or the way they entertained their guests. Then let them talk some more. Listen. Savor. You're hearing the voice of the past that will be gone all too soon. Sit in their midst and soak it up. You may find that you enjoy it so much you want to make it a regular part of your life.

Child, Maiden, Lover, Mother, Crone, the circle of woman-knowledge is eternal and ever growing. Listen to it. Keep it going.

☙

Chapter 3

CROWNING GLORY

Your Hair from Conditioning to Covering

Listen,
Ostrich plumes differ
From chicken feathers.
OKOT P'BITEK
Song of Lawino

THE DANDELION COIFFURE of a young woman strolling through the Dan Tokpa market in Cotonou, Benin; the "mud-caked" hair of a child scampering through the twisting alleyways of Fès el-Bali in Morocco; the lustrous single sable braid swaying rhythmically down the back of a *bharata natya* dancer; the intricate cornrows that peek out from under a Senegalese coquette's *mousor* or head scarf; the tightly pulled bun of a Chinese grandmother—hair is a major part of our first impression of any woman.

Hair is perhaps the most loaded subject in the entire world of beauty. Crowning glory or crown of pain? Hair has been a bane and a blessing for women of color for centuries. The bane part comes when western European canons of beauty overlay majority-world realities and generations of black, yellow, and brown women rely on all sorts of methods to fight the natural flow of their hair. The blessing part comes when the hair is allowed to be itself and reveals itself to be healthy, vibrant, strong, and resilient, as indeed the women are themselves.

Recently, I attended a one-day symposium given by students at the university at which I teach. My professional demeanor was reduced to a war whoop of victory when one student read a paper on racial attitudes in the work of a Latina author. Her title for the paper? "Pelo Bueno/Pelo Malo" (Good hair/bad hair). The succinct four-word title summed up the method by which many were judged in my not-so-distant childhood. It also revealed that the happenings that I had thought of as personal were indeed universal.

The mere thought of hair takes me back to the kitchen. In wafts the particular smell of a blue glob of Posner's bergamot on the back of a brown hand intermingled with that of a hot straightening comb. I think of childhood agony sitting between my mother's legs as she valiantly attempted to "tame" my thick and unruly hair. The taming of my hair was perhaps a metaphor for the taming of me. It was only as I got older that I realized that what was a profound personal memory was actually a racial memory; generations of African American women have bonded over hair.

Problems have been discussed, dissected, debated, and resolved over hot oil treatments. Lost or left or lackluster lovers were mourned while the hot comb flew, and aching muscles and tired bodies were soothed and smoothed as caring black hands rubbed and shampooed away the pains of generations. Heartaches and unhappiness were washed down the drain with the rinse water. This was the experience of African American women. Those of Latina and Asian descent, while not always shaped by the same experiences, were, in the twentieth century, nonetheless shaped by the same craving for the long strawberry-blond ringlets of Boticelli's Venus, or the sheet of raven hair of Morticia Addams, or the blond locks of Shirley Temple.

Over the years, I have found my own experiences mirrored in those of friends around the world. Michele Rakotosan, a playwright from Madagascar, remembered being taunted for her lightly curled hair, which was too "African" for her mother's taste, while Christina Ng in Singapore confided that she had spent her childhood praying for more curl to her hair so that she could wear Western styles. All three of us were unwary victims of Europe's aesthetic colonization of the world. Interestingly, we had all arrived at our own personal peace with our crowning glory, realizing that our hair is like a good friend. As with all friends, you must occasionally adjust to its temperaments and its tantrums, but you really love it deep down because it is a part of you.

Coming to grips with your hair is a sign of maturity, and once you do, you'll realize that hair and hair care have long been at the center of women's friendship and women's bonding. In Mali and other parts of West Africa, women enjoy their time together in courtyards called *keur awa* (Eve's courts). These traditional beauty parlors are a refuge from the rigors of the world. There is no more soothing touch than that of a loved one combing or brushing our hair. Try it with a friend: sit at her feet, hand her the brush, and give yourself up to the rhythmic stroking of your hair. . . . Heaven!

Hairstyles are rife with herstory and meaning. They can indicate a woman's age and status in the community. They can tell of lineage and speak eloquently of class and caste. The act of covering or not covering the head can in itself be an act of defiance or of immeasurable coquetry, while the item with which the hair is covered can speak of family or religious background. In West Africa, a young woman's hairstyle may show her age and family lineage and even celebrate local events. In the late 1950s, when Nigeria's featherweight boxer Hogan Kid-Bassey won his championship in Los Angeles, there was a hairstyle called "Los." Other Nigerian styles have been called "Don't touch; he's crazy," "Eko Bridge" (after a noted Lagos bridge), and "pineapple."

In Senegal, young unmarried girls wear their hair uncovered, revealing imaginative cornrow hairstyles with special names like *"tati panier"* and *"adra"* that change with the whims of fashion. Their older, married sisters have their hair braided in intricate, more mature styles, but they hide their tresses under their *mousor* as a sign that they are married women. When they are widowed, part of the attendant ritual is the ceremonial unbraiding and, in orthodox cases, the shaving of the widow's hair as a sign that she will shun vanity until her period of mourning is over.

In the Malagasy Republic, the women of the Betsileo people wear individual braids that are shaped to look like flat curls. Once finished, the coiffure is coated with a mixture of animal fat and honey called *tavo*, which hardens and fixes the hair. If a woman is widowed while wearing the hairstyle, the hair is shaved in such a way that the hardened hair can be maintained and worn as a wig once her mourning period is over.

In parts of India, a young woman signals her coming of age when she goes from wearing the two braids of childhood to wearing a single one down her back. In Japan, geisha wear different styles and even different wigs to celebrate holidays and signal special events. In other parts of the Far East, hairdressing ceremonies accompany traditional weddings. In the past, women like the amahs of China and Hong Kong and the *sam sui* of Singapore underwent a hair-binding ceremony during which they took vows and pledged to remain single. Japanese brides dress in the traditional manner and wear their hair or wigs in elaborate upswept hairstyles that are adorned with ornaments of peach blossoms and silk ribbons called *shimada.*

Hair ornaments are, in fact, an important part of the hairstyles of the women of the majority world. Flowers, both real and artificial, have long blossomed on the heads of women in tropical climates, whether the delicate *shimada* of cherry or peach blossoms in the glossy hair of a traditional Japanese bride, the tiny orchids encircling the knot of hair at the nape of a Singaporean woman's neck, the hibiscus smiling out from the dark curly locks of a Caribbean woman, or even Billie Holiday's gardenia. Combs in every material from shell, ivory, bone, and lacquered wood to antique tortoiseshell also enhance traditional hairdos. The Peul/Fulani women of Mali adorn their hair with heavy beads of African amber called copal and may even have so many woven into their intricate braids that they seem to be an amber cap. In northern Senegal, gold or gold-dipped base metal called *sassal* is formed into trefoils, stars, and other designs that are then sewn into braided hair. Brightly colored ribbons are braided into the ebony tresses of many Mexican Indian women. Feathers, beads, and more, so much more, are incorporated into women's hairstyles around the world.

Hair and ornaments to adorn it do not tell the whole story. Hair coverings are important, too—so important, in fact, that in antebellum New Orleans, sumptuary laws defined what could and could not be worn by women of color. Because women of color were thought to be too alluring, they were forbidden to wear hats and forced to wear head ties called *tignons*. (The flair for fashion of nineteenth-century octoroons and quadroons was legendary and a sore point among the European women of the town.) In later years, the head tie was thought of as an object of derision, a covering for Aunt Jemima's head. However, the fine, colored Creoles took a cue from their sisters in Martinique and Guadeloupe and created head ties of such beauty and intricacy that they by far eclipsed the mere hats of the European women!

Head ties are traditional to much of the African Atlantic world and hark back to parts of western African where the tying of one's head signals adulthood for women. This language of the head tie is still seen in Afro-Brazilian religious communities and in the traditional dress of the French-speaking Caribbean, where head ties from brightly printed Indian madras fabric can indicate a woman's social and marital status. The African Atlantic world is not alone in its reverence for head ties and hair ornaments.

Think of twentieth-century artist Frida Kahlo's inventive ways with yarn, fabric, and traditional Mexican headwear.

There is no monolithic hair with a capital *H* for women of color. Hair textures and types are as varied as elsewhere. Hair ranges from ruler-straight to tightly curled kinks and may be oily, dry, or any number of combinations and permutations in between. Texture may be baby-hair fine or steel-wool coarse. Whatever yours is, love it! Enjoy it! It is a living witness to your personal history, a living link with your past—and for that alone it deserves to be well cared for. It's also one of the first things about you that people notice, so make it a positive one.

Experiment with your hair. Challenge yourself to an occasional half-hour in front of the mirror with comb, brush, and hairpins. Try a new style. Ask yourself what is your biggest hair challenge and what is your biggest hair plus. Then work with them both until you're no longer afraid of or mad at your hair. Ask your girlfriends what are their hair challenges, and have a good time swapping "hair-raising" tales of childhood traumas and bad haircuts. Then shampoo them all down the drain metaphorically, and literally. Start loving your hair. It's one of the steps to loving yourself in all that you are and in all that you can be.

HEAD-CLEARING RITUAL

As with all beauty, hair beauty begins on the inside. In this case, cleanse your head of negativity before you begin to work on your hair. To the Yoruba of southwestern Nigeria, the head or *ori* is the seat of the soul. It is necessary, therefore, to nourish, strengthen, and cleanse it regularly. A friend who follows the ways of the African gods in the New World taught me a Yoruba head-cleaning exercise. It can cleanse negativity and help when you're troubled, or it can simply help you attain calm and peace of mind. I've tried it on numerous occasions: I can't say whether it's the slow, steady, deliberate, ritually prescribed movements or the fact that you're concentrating on ridding yourself of the problem, but it works.

Once you have decided to try this, proceed in complete silence. Turn off music and all intruding sound and concentrate on yourself. First, find a quiet, peaceful corner of your living space. Wash your hands. (If you are not near water, find a calm spot and make Lady Macbeth–like washing motions with your hands.) Return to your calm spot and shake out your hands as though drying them by flinging the water away from you. Then, starting at the center of your forehead, using both hands like wands, move each hand outward toward your ears. When the hands reach your ears, shake them vigorously, as though shaking them dry. Beginning once again at the middle of your forehead, move your hands up just over the top of your head and down to the nape of your neck. Continue with the hands moving simultaneously until your hands have reached your clavicles. Then shake them as though drying them. Finally—this cleanses your aura—start at the middle of your forehead and repeat the second movement, lifting the hands higher to cleanse the air around your head. Be sure to flick your hands in the drying motion at the end of each pass; with this action you are "throwing off" the problem and the negativity. When you've completed the three phases of the process, sit down and remain quiet and still for fifteen minutes or longer while still concentrating on your problem or your thoughts. Then resume business as usual. You'll be surprised. You'll feel more at peace with yourself. Try it; it's cheaper than a drink or a shrink and better for you than a pill. Inner head cleansed, it's time to proceed to the care of your hair.

A note from the Far East: Hair care begins under the skin with what you eat. In Japan, they eat kelp and seafood regularly to promote hair growth and to enhance the glossiness of the hair. You can do the same by eating green leafy vegetables for their vitamin E and by following a well-balanced diet that gives you all the vitamins and minerals you need. Watch your diet, and soon folks will be watching your hair.

CONDITIONING

Condition—it's a magic command in hair care today. Everyone is looking for the correct conditioner to promote abundant hair growth and clean, healthy hair. What's surprising is that conditioners aren't new. Cleopatra reportedly used bear grease or natural lanolin to make her hair grow, while the Queen of Sheba applied henna to give her hair color and make it manageable. Josephine Baker used egg yolks to condition her hair and the whites to keep her spit curls in place.

—————————— ✦ ——————————

Mama's Hot Oil Treatment

Years ago, before the general public became aware of the need to condition their hair and hair-care product lines expanded to include all sorts of conditioners, my mother used to give me hot oil treatments for my dry scalp. She would melt a little Vaseline in a saucepan until it was warm (*not hot*—you don't want to scorch your scalp!). Then she would section my hair and, with a cotton ball, apply the tepid liquid Vaseline to my scalp. This was a special treat and an easy one to duplicate.

4 tablespoons Vaseline petroleum jelly

1 small saucepan

10 or more cotton balls

Place the Vaseline in the saucepan and warm it over low heat until it liquefies. Watch it carefully, as Vaseline is flammable. Also be careful not to get it too hot; if this happens, let it cool off before you use it.

Section the hair. Make one long part from front to back, another from ear to ear, and keep dividing until you have eight sections. Using the cotton balls, apply the warm Vaseline to the parts. Then massage the entire head with the balls of your fingers. Leave the oil on for an hour—or overnight, if possible. (If overnight, tie your head in a towel so that the oil doesn't damage your pillowcase.) Then shampoo as usual. You'll find that your hair looks more lustrous and feels silkier.

If you'd like to add some extra zing to Mama's Hot Oil Treatment, proceed according to the instructions. Then instead of simply washing out the Vaseline or going to sleep, wrap a steaming-hot towel around your head. The hot towel will help the scalp absorb the oil. Apply the hot towels three times at twenty-minute intervals; then allow your hair to rest. Shampoo and proceed as usual.

Oils and oil treatments like my mother's are used by women of color all around the world. In Guyana, they use warmed castor oil to promote hair growth. In Mexico, women swear by the hot oil bath they give their hair. Caribbean women use a variation of this same treatment with coconut oil. In India, they use gingelly oil (sesame oil); in Tunisia, olive oil and sweet almond oil; and in parts of West Africa, *karite* or shea butter, a natural vegetable butter, for the same treatments. At the Floating Market in Curaçao, a green oil from Venezuela, sold in old pint rum bottles, can sometimes be found among the fruits and vegetables. It's avocado oil, and it's a hair-care wonder. When it is used instead of Vaseline in a hot oil bath, the hair seems to become particularly soft and manageable, and the avocado oil even prevents tangling. Many of the oils used by women of color in this manner are obtainable at health-food stores.

Shea butter is another particularly wonderful find. It's used for all manner of beauty rituals in West Africa and has even been discovered by European trichologists like René Furterer. Said to promote hair growth and hair strength, it is also a detangler. It can be used as a body rub and is thought to prevent stretch marks (more about that in another chapter). Shea butter, though, is not the only one. Castor oil, sesame oil, jojoba oil, olive oil, coconut oil, and sweet almond oil can all be used in this manner. If you use an oil like sweet almond oil, you can add the extra element of fragrance by mixing it with a few drops of your favorite essential oil before applying.

Ixtapan de la Sal is a wonderful spa outside Mexico City where you can be pampered and beautified to your heart's delight. Built on mineral springs, the spa has been a place of revitalization since Aztec times. It's only natural after that long a history that they should have some excellent hair-conditioning hints.

Aceites Mezcladas a la Ixtapan
(Mixed oils Ixtapan style)

The spa at Ixtapan has an oil treatment similar to my mother's. When I spent some time there, my dry, overprocessed hair drank up the oil treatment like a balm for its soul. Ixtapan's mixture of oils in its hot oil treatment is a well-guarded secret. As a treatment for extremely dry hair, my version works almost as well, though. It can also serve as a summer treat for dry or sun-parched hair.

¼ cup lemon oil   ¼ cup castor oil

¼ cup almond oil   ¼ cup olive oil

1 yard plastic wrap

Separate the hair into eight sections and apply the oil mixture with cotton balls. Wrap the hair in plastic wrap, or use a shower cap, and sit under a warm hair dryer for forty-five minutes. If you have a heat cap, you can omit the plastic wrap. Alternately, the oil mixture can be left on overnight. In that case, wrap the hair in a towel to avoid soiling your bed linen. Whichever method you use, when finished, shampoo and proceed as usual.

Mayo Conditioner

African American women have traditionally turned to what is at hand for many of their beauty practices. This is true also with hair. Here, they had no farther to look than the mayonnaise jar. The summer-salad staple is an excellent hair conditioner as well. After all, when homemade, it's only an emulsion of oil and egg. What could be better for soothing dry, damaged hair?

4 tablespoons homemade or commercial mayonnaise
1 yard plastic wrap

Section the hair. Apply the mayonnaise to the sections. Massage the scalp vigorously. Wrap the hair in plastic wrap and leave it on for one hour. Shampoo and proceed with styling the hair as usual.

Not all women of color have dry hair, although it is fairly common because of climatic conditions in the areas in which we live. There are also solutions for oily-hair problems. Women of color traditionally use natural products in their beauty regimens. One of the New World items that is a favorite in tropical countries is the avocado. In many parts of the world, avocado trees line the countryside and the avocados are simply there for the picking. They're used for everything from soothing roughened skin to conditioning the hair.

Marlene's Avocado Magic

Here's a secret that I got from Marlene, a Trinidadian friend. Marlene is a grandmother, but you would never guess it from looking at her. Her complexion is wonderful and her hair is lustrous and soft. She made me rethink my whole idea of how a grandmother should look. She's a living embodiment of the African American saying that "good black don't crack." If she uses avocados, they're worth a try by the rest of us. Here's what she does.

½ overripe avocado

Take half of a very ripe avocado and mash it in a blender at low speed. Apply the pulp to the hair, massaging it in to spread it evenly. Let the avocado mixture remain on the hair and scalp for half an hour; then wash it out with a mild shampoo and proceed as usual.

Moroccan women with oily hair swear by the natural conditioner called *gassouhl,* which can be found in large baskets in Moroccan markets. If I hadn't heard its praises sung so often, I would certainly not have tried it, for it looks like dried chips of mud or something else singularly unmentionable. It is used like henna in that it is mixed with water and applied to the hair, left for one hour, and then washed out. *Gassouhl* is not readily available in the United States, but it can be found in some stores in Arab neighborhoods or through mail-order sources (see appendix A). It's an excellent conditioner, and I've heard Moroccan women with *dry* hair bemoaning the fact that there's nothing like it for them.

Henna is a hair-care herb that has been known since ancient times. Prepared from the cut or ground leaves of a North African plant, *Lawsonia inermis,* henna can be used to dye the hair various shades of red or black, or simply to condition it, as with colorless henna. The henna coats the hair shaft and temporarily gives the hair more body. It is applied by women in Morocco and Tunisia before they head off to the *hammam* or steam bath. Anyone who has walked through the twisty alleyways of the residential areas of the medina in Marrakech or Fès has seen young girls and older women scurrying along looking as though they had mud packs on their heads. The mud is henna, and women of the Arab world swear by it.

⚜

Khadijah's Henna Treatment

Khadijah was the first to teach me how to use henna, so I've named the treatment for her. Although henna is complicated to apply and still has the stigma of leaving hair flaming red (think Lucille Ball and all her Technicolor Lucy Hennaed hair jokes), if you're careful, follow the directions, and do not attempt to use henna on blond, gray, or white hair, you'll be pleased with the lustrous results. Here's how Khadijah does it, but you should follow the directions on whatever henna you purchase.

½ pound colorless henna

1 pint hot water

Rubber gloves

A clean white cloth or towel that you don't mind permanently dirtying

Henna must be applied to already-shampooed hair. The night before, do a skin-patch test on your arm. Mix a small amount of the henna with water and apply it to a patch of skin about one inch square on your arm where it won't be visible. Leave it uncovered and allow it to dry for four hours. Watch it closely to see if you have any itching or burning, or develop any redness or other unusual reactions. If not, test a small strand of hair first to avoid any unpleasant surprises. Snip a small amount of hair and tie it with a thread. Soak the sample in the henna you plan to use. If you're happy with the results, proceed.

Mix the henna and water together in a nonreactive bowl. Use a wooden chopstick or spoon to stir the mixture (a metal spoon will cause a chemical reaction). With rubber gloves on, rub the henna mixture into the hair as evenly as possible. Be careful not to allow the mixture to drip because henna is a dye and if it drips, you're dyed.

Cover your hair with plastic wrap, or a used shower cap, wrap the towel around the plastic, then sit in a warm place. Allow the mixture to remain on the hair for the prescribed time. This can be anything from five minutes to an hour, and it is not un-heard of for Moroccan women to leave their henna packs on overnight. Since there are various types of henna on the market, it's best to check and follow the individual package directions. Whatever the directions, when the henna is ready, you'll rinse it out and be conditioned. If you've used red or black henna, you'll be dyed as well.

In Morocco, women add other herbs to henna to produce variations on its basic colors of red and black. Indigo is occasionally used to give the hair blue highlights. A Caribbean hairdresser told me that she mixes in a bit of rum for a deep brown hue. Once you've mastered the basic treatment, you may want to try a little judicious experimentation for a color that is uniquely yours. Just remember the strand test, so you don't end up looking like an or-ange dandelion.

❊

Indian Henna Conditioner

Henna conditioners are also used in India, where women add a bit of well-steeped tea to the henna mixture. They also make an excel-lent henna-based conditioner for dry hair.

¼ cup colorless henna

½ cup plain yogurt

2 teaspoons freshly squeezed lime juice

Mix the ingredients together in a nonreactive bowl. Section the hair into eight segments and apply the henna mixture to the sectioned hair. Leave the henna mixture on for about half an hour (again, this time will depend on the type of henna purchased), then wash out.

An Egyptian friend added yet another possibility to the henna conditioners by mentioning a recipe similar to the Indian one, except that she uses an egg yolk and two tablespoons of yogurt instead of the lime juice and yogurt.

CLEANSING

Conditioning is the first step to attaining luxuriant, healthy hair, but cleansing is a continual part of the process. The Yoruba of southwestern Nigeria and neighboring Benin swear by their *osé dudu* or black soap made from palm oil, palm nut kernels, and ash. The soap is sold in grainy dark-brown balls in the traditional markets like the Adjara Yoruba market, outside Porto-Novo. The soap looks as though it should be harsh, but it is remarkably gentle—it is used for bathing babies and considered by many to be excellent for the scalp.

Native Americans had many recipes for hair care and taught the early colonists a thing or two about general hygiene. The Kiowa used the root of the soap plant mixed with water as a shampoo. They found that the mixture was not only good for cleansing; it was also effective against dandruff and worked wonders on an irritated scalp.

In the American Southwest, chlorogalum, a member of the lily family, was used as a shampoo, and the Hopi found that the sap of the yucca plant did the trick. Because these plants are usually available only in their growing areas, it is difficult for them to catch on elsewhere. Another Native American plant, soapwort root, though, can be obtained almost everywhere, either from health-food stores or through mail-order sources.

Soapwort root, which belongs to the carnation family, will lather when put into water. It has been used to cleanse fabric since ancient Egyptian days and is still used by those who clean and maintain antique clothing. The mild sudsing properties of the plant make it a wonderfully delicate shampoo. It has been used as such by Native Americans since before the arrival of the early colonists.

——————————————— ✵ ———————————————

Native American Hair Wash

⅛ ounce soapwort root
1¼ pints boiling water

Crush the soapwort root. Infuse it in hot water by pouring the boiling water over the soapwort root chips and letting the mixture steep as you would tea. The mixture should steep for half an hour. Then, strain the mixture through a sieve to remove the soapwort root chips and use the liquid to shampoo hair.

You can also prepare your own mild shampoo from pure castile soap and scent it by adding sage, rosemary, chamomile, or lavender flowers and a few drops of essential oil.

——————————————— ✵ ———————————————

Castile Cleanser

½ pint water
¼ cup lavender blossoms (undyed)
4 drops lavender essential oil
¼ cup grated castile soap

Place the water in a small saucepan and bring it to a boil. Then lower the heat and add the lavender and the lavender oil and allow the mixture to simmer for fifteen or twenty minutes. Strain the water through cheesecloth to remove the herbs, and add the grated castile soap to the water. Place the mixture in a jar to use immediately or in the near future. You can vary the herbs and the oil as your whimsy takes you.

If you have neither the time nor the inclination to prepare your own shampoo, you can still join in the fun by adding ingredients to already purchased pure shampoos. Beginning with a castile shampoo, add:

Molasses for hair vitamins
Egg yolks for body
Coal tar for dandruff treatment
Creosote for dandruff treatment
Sweet almond oil for conditioning and detangling
Essential oils for fragrance

Take the time to experiment a bit. As long as what you're adding is basically healthy and in small amounts proportionate to the amount of shampoo, you're only helping yourself and personalizing the shampoo to your individual needs.

Dry Shampoo

Occasionally, there's just not enough time to shampoo and you're faced with the choice of wearing a turban or a paper bag. A dry-shampoo tip comes from traditional African Americans, who used it to shampoo the hair of the sick. It simply involves sprinkling a bit of cornmeal or hominy grits onto the scalp and then brushing the hair vigorously. The dry ingredient will help remove hair oil and other debris, and the hair will be cleaner. Needless to say, these quick-shampoo methods are to be used when water is not feasible or practical. Otherwise, shampoo regularly.

Mom's Quick Perk-Up

My mother, bless her heart, taught me this trick years ago. Take a brush and force the bristles through an old stocking or a section cut from a pair of old panty hose. (At last, there's a use for old panty hose!) Brush your hair normally. You'll be surprised at the "ick" that you'll see when you remove the panty hose section. Rewrap the brush in another section and continue until your hair is presentable. This is one of Mama's lifesavers that really helps in a pinch.

RINSES

Women of color have long been aware that a finishing rinse leaves their hair smoother and more lustrous. In China, cedrela, otherwise known as "stinky cedar," is a main source of scent. When it is infused and applied to the hair as a rinse, it is thought to promote hair growth. In the Philippines, women steep a few blades of aloe in cold water and use the water as a tonic rinse. And in ancient Arabia, the brewed peel of the quince was used as a lotion on the hair of women and on the tails and manes of the famous Arabian horses. (You can't get a better recommendation than that!) In some cases, though, the simplest rinses are the best. From time to time, I still return to the traditional vinegar rinse. It not only smooths the hair; it also restores the hair's natural acid mantle.

Traditional Vinegar Rinse

¼ cup distilled vinegar
2 pints warm water

Mix the vinegar and water together in a small bowl and pour it over the head as the final rinse. This will also help to untangle hair.

The recipe can be jazzed up by adding various herbs to the vinegar. Simply add the herbs to the vinegar, allow them to steep for the allotted time, strain them out, and then proceed as in the basic rinse.

FOR DANDRUFF

Simmer 1 teaspoon of nettles in the vinegar for thirty minutes.

FOR LIGHT HAIR

Simmer 1 teaspoon of chamomile in the vinegar for thirty minutes. This will slightly lighten the color of hair.

FOR DARK HAIR

Simmer 1 teaspoon of sage in the vinegar for thirty minutes. This will slightly darken the hair.

FOR SUN STREAKS

Instead of ¼ cup of vinegar, use ¼ cup of freshly squeezed lemon juice. The lemon juice will give the hair a fresh citrusy scent and will lighten it slightly when exposed to sunlight.

Note: These rinses are for hair that has *not* been processed. Don't try them with hair that has been bleached, permed, or otherwise tampered with, for the chemical reaction of the rinse with the hair may not be what you wish!

STYLING

Though women of color spend much of their hair beauty time attending to the conditioning and cleanliness of their hair, their ultimate glory is in the styling. This holds true for styles ranging from the complicated cornrow and wrapped hairdos of West Africa to the sophisticated buns and chignons of the Far East. In many areas, style attains such importance that it is not only adornment, it is also totemic.

In Senegal, as in many West African nations, when a girl begins to braid her hair, it is a sign that she is an adolescent. The tufts of her childhood style will depend on her ethnic group in some areas and may be as much an identifying mark as her name. West African styles have caught on with African American women, and any walk through an African American neighborhood will reveal a number of beauty parlors and hair-braiding salons offering a mind-boggling multiplicity of hairstyles. Hair braiding and cornrowing are so popular that they have even been adopted by Europeans on summer vacation. Braiding centers have sprung up in Ocho Rios and Montego Bay on Jamaica's north coast and on other islands, and for many returning from vacation, hair full of braids and beads is as much a sign of having been away as returning with a tan.

In Africa, there is a communal feeling to hair care. Friends braid and style each other's hair at home and spend long hours sitting, chatting, and finishing intricate hairstyles. Some of today's deceptively simple-looking styles can take as many as ten hours to execute, while the complex ones can take two days or more. My first African cornrow style took ten hours to complete in a *keur awa* in Dakar, Senegal. A *keur awa* is an interior courtyard where hair braiders and other traditional beauticians work. I almost balked when I realized that the hairdresser was making the myriad parts in my hair with an ice pick, but I persevered. Theodora, my good friend from Benin, spent the full day with me, bringing me food, gossiping, and keeping me from being bored and becoming cranky. I loved the braids, the convenience of not having to wonder if my hair was right in the morning, the ability to go swimming without a second thought as to how much time hair drying and arranging would take before the next activity, and, most of all, the feeling of always being well kempt. However, when my parts began to get a bit fuzzy after a few weeks, and when I got tired of the same style all the time, they had to come out. Little did I realize when it took ten hours getting them in that it would take me more than four hours to get them out. Just as I was about to chuck it all, give up, and get a razor, Theodora came to my rescue again. She also gave me a great hint for removing the cornrows.

Thea's Braid Secret

1 porcupine quill
(or 1 small-gauge plastic knitting needle)

Insert the pointy end of the quill between the hair and the scalp at the top of the braid and gently lift, loosening the hair slightly. Then, beginning at the bottom of each braid, use the porcupine quill to undo the braid from the bottom up. This must be done oh-so-carefully so that hair is not pulled out by the roots. It's time-consuming, but it works.

SPECIAL HAIR PROBLEMS

We all have special hair problems, from split ends to bald spots. While they are for the most part personal pains, they are also universal. The first recipe for baldness on record was prepared for a woman—Ses, Queen Mother of His Majesty the King of Upper and Lower Egypt, Teta—over five thousand years ago. It was prepared from toes of a dog, date refuse, and an ass's hoof. The Ebers Papyrus abounds with remedies for baldness and potions designed to promote hair growth, including some that seem remarkably contemporary—like linseed crushed in oil and rubbed on the scalp and castor oil baths for the hair. Others call for more esoteric ingredients: lion and hippopotamus fat, blood from the neck of the gabu bird, and gazelle's dung.

Ses was also one of the first to use hair dye and one of the first people on record as having used henna. Today, traditional women in parts of Tunisia dye their hair with henna or with a mixture called *mardouma* prepared from galls, cloves, and copper sulfate. The galls and cloves are burned together and then pounded in a mortar, after which the powdered copper sulfate is added. These ingredients are mixed with water and the concoction simmered over a low flame until it becomes a black liquid. *Mardouma* and other black hair dyes come in handy in Tunisia because all traditional brides, be they blonds or redheads, dye their hair black. The dark hair is thought to be particularly provocative for its contrast with the pale white makeup also worn on their wedding days.

The Egyptian queen Ses may not have had split ends, but Dorotea, my friend from the Dominican Republic, does, and she taught me a trick for getting rid of them.

Dorotea's Split End Trick

1 corncob

Scorch the corncob over a flame; then use it to brush the ends of your hair. The cob will remove the split ends.

ADORNING

Hairstyles, no matter how seemingly simple, are usually decorated by women of color. Whether it's a hibiscus flower just picked from a nearby bush, an intricately carved jade comb, or a crown of amber and gold beads, a hair ornament adds that little something extra that says "I am me," we personalize our coiffures. Traditional Japanese brides wear hair ornaments of tortoiseshell. The beads, hair terminations, and clips that are sewn onto African American women's cornrows are descendants and adaptations of the cowrie shells, beads, and golden ornaments that adorn many traditional African styles. Ribbons and yarn added to braids are typical of many Mexican women, and around the world, pins, combs, and ornaments of all sizes, shapes, materials, and colors appear.

One of the simplest and most elegant ways to enhance any hairstyle is with flowers. It is a universal method of ornamentation. Fresh flowers are best because they will not only decorate but also add fragrance to your hair. In ancient China, heavily oiled or pomaded hair was arranged into elegant buns and styles that imitated everything from teapot handles to butterflies. All were adorned with flowers, which were sometimes placed inside small water-filled tubes hidden in the hair to maintain their freshness.

When you next fix your hair for an evening, try arranging a fresh spray of baby's breath around a bun and see what a difference it will make. An ordinary style can be transformed into something extraordinary. Also think of the coquettish placement of a single flower like Billie Holiday's gardenia. Let your imagination be your guide. But don't overwhelm your hairstyle and begin to look like an ambulatory garden; think small and simple. Be sure to choose a hardy flower that will last for a while; baby's breath is perfect for this reason. Nothing is better than fresh flowers in the hair, but nothing looks worse than a wilting rose in a hairstyle. One way to beat this is to use artificial flowers, but you won't have the benefit of natural fragrance. Tacky, you say. Not so if the flower is a single lovely, elegant silk blossom. I purchased a fabric sunflower in a boutique in Jamaica that has fooled more than one person into commenting on the fresh flower that I wore in my hair. I, in fact, liked it so much that on a return trip, I bought another one.

Silk flowers do not compare to fresh ones, but they have the elegance of silk, the allure of a rainbow of colors, and the added plus that they will not wilt. A single silk tiger lily tucked alongside an elegant bun or French twist can make a knockout evening style that's sophisticated and savvy. You can even scent it to match your perfume or spray it with a version of its own fragrance for the added plus of scent.

Fragrant, scented hair is an idea that Senegalese coquettes called *diryankes* have developed into a fine art. They perfume their hair, not with rinses, or even with scented oils, but rather with the smoky, sensuous fragrance of their own personally prepared incense called *thiouraye.*

·※·

Thiane's Thiouraye Secret

When drying her hair, Thiane, my Senegalese friend, places her incense burner of *thiouraye* nearby. The smoky scent permeates the room and everything in it, including Thiane's hair and clothing. By preparing her own incense mixture, she is able to have a distinctive scent that is hers alone.

Try this with your own prepared *thiouraye* (see chapter 8) or with a few incense sticks of your choice. Leave them burning nearby as you blow-dry your hair or allow the hair to dry naturally and absorb the scent.

TOPPING IT OFF

Head ties and head wraps are an important part of the dress of the exotic world. The same Malian woman who will spend two days in a *keur awa* getting her hair braided will then spend more time tying her head wrap into a style so intricate that it will almost be a hat. The same grace with tying fabric into headwear came over with the Africans in the holds of slave ships and blossomed forth once again in the madras head ties of Martinique and Guadeloupe, the turbans of Salvador da Bahia, Brazil, the *tignons* of New Orleans, and, yes, Aunt Jemima's bandana. Each had a meaning and an importance. In Martinique, there was even a language of the head tie. Madras turbans with one point heading skyward meant that the young woman was single; two signaled that she was married; three indicated that she was married but still looking; and four meant that she was a *matadore,* one of the infamous courtesans who made provocation of the male of the species their amply rewarded life's work. In Bahia, in the Afro-Brazilian Candomblé houses of worship, the way a turban was tied indicated whether a practitioner was a votary of a male or a female *orișa*. Studies even suggest that in colonial times, slaves could identify one another by the design of their head ties.

Recently, while spending some time at a *terreiro* in Brazil, I astonished the women at a gathering by knowing exactly how to tie a head tie in their traditional manner. How did I know? I don't know; perhaps it's an atavism that lies dormant within the hands of all African women in the diaspora. Whatever your race, knowing how to tie a turban can be very useful. They're perfect for "bad hair days," excellent for surprise company, and a great way to cheat after a day at the beach.

Aunt Jemima's Bandana

Now you leave Aunt Jemima alone. She's on that box because she made the best pancakes around. That she didn't get royalties for it and that she had no say wasn't her fault. She was a more reliable cook, though, than many today. How do you know? Because she took care to tie her hair up so that it wouldn't get into the food. Take a hint from her when you have housework to do or when you're seriously cooking.

1 thirty-six-inch scarf or square of cloth

Take the scarf and fold it into a triangle. With the point of the triangle facing your forehead, grasp the two long ends and tie them over the point. Take the point of the triangle and fold it backwards over the knot, tucking it in. Voilà, your hair is out of your face and you're ready to get to work. If you want to give Aunt Jemima some payback, wear a silk-scarf version of this head tie when you are going out.

Bahian Turban

In Bahian Candomblés, this turban or *torco* is tied from a long rectangle of white cloth whose ends are embroidered with designs that may be symbolic of the wearer's *orisa*. Daughters of Yemanja will have flying fish or starfish, and daughters of Osun may have butterflies or mirrors. The turban is simple to wear and easy to tie.

1 long, narrow scarf or a long rectangle of cloth that is at least one and a half yards long

With one end of the scarf in each hand, hold the scarf behind your head. Bring the edges of the scarf toward your face, cross them over, and return them to the back of the turban, where you tuck them in. Depending on the width of your scarf, you'll have either a headband turban that will keep your hair neatly in place in the front while leaving it out in the back, or a full head cover. This turban works best if you use a cotton or rayon fabric that can be slightly pulled to make it fit snugly.

Chapter 4

BEST FACE FORWARD

A Radiant Complexion, Clear Eyes, and a Fresh Mouth

1. Behold thou art fair, my love: behold thou art fair. . . .
2. Thy teeth are like a flock of sheep that are even shorn, which came up from the washing whereof every one bears twins, and none is barren among them.
3. Thy lips are like a thread of scarlet, and thy speech is comely: thy temples are like a piece of pomegranate within thy locks.

SONG OF SONGS 1:1–4

WHETHER OF TRANSLUCENT-LOOKING alabaster hue or deep aubergine-tinted black, a clear complexion is a sign of great beauty throughout the world. Women of traditional cultures value their complexions and usually have excellent ones because of simple, basic skin-care methods that are not counteracted by heavy makeup and diets of "junk" foods. Over the centuries, travelers have marveled at the wonderful matte complexions that the women of Haiti and Martinique maintain, the ocher smoothness of the Masai women of East Africa, the seemingly poreless look of a plum-tinted Senegalese woman, or the pearly ivory visage of a Singaporean Nonya woman.

The methods used to maintain these complexions may be as simple as a dab of coconut oil or as complex as the formula for Royal Concubine

Radiant Beauty Cream, which Asian women can pick up at Vera's World in Hong Kong. This cream, produced in the People's Republic of China, contains ginseng, pulverized white jade, and pearl powder, the traditional Chinese ingredient for smooth, translucent skin. Coconut oils and pearl powders, though, are only the tip of the facial iceberg.

Egg-white facial masques have been used as far back in time as ancient Egypt. Honey is a natural moisturizer as well, and it's very easy to imagine some beekeeper's wife of yore slathering her face with honey with luminous results. Avocados have been not only a sustaining food in the tropical world for centuries, but also a well-kept beauty secret in Latin America since pre-Columbian times. For centuries, women in China, Turkey, and North Africa have used henna on faces as well as on hands and hair.

In parts of China, the aesthetic calls for a face as round as the moon, while among several Native American groups the forehead was flattened as a sign of beauty. Around the world, tattoos, paints, rouges, and more have enhanced the face that we put forward to the world. The fact that our main organ of communication, the mouth, is set in the face makes it the center of our beauty universe. Of equal importance with the mouth are the eyes. They are indeed the windows of the soul, and in some countries may be the only part of a woman that is visible. As bodies became covered and adorned, the face remained in many cultures the last bastion of beauty originality.

Eye makeup is probably one of the oldest forms of body painting. It goes back well beyond ancient Egypt. The Egyptians, though, were masters of eye makeup and derived many eye-painting techniques that we still use today. In ancient Egypt, eye paint was also medicinal. It was designed to protect the eyes from the sun. The paint was prepared by grinding raw materials like antimony, oxides of copper, iron, manganese, and other ingredients on a stone slab. The powders were then placed in hollow reed containers or in alabaster jars to be stored until used. When the woman was ready for her toilette, the containers were set out and the pigments were then mixed with oils or animal fats. At other times, the powders were applied alone over a base or ointment, like our eye shadow. The underside of the eyes was painted with a dark green cosmetic, and the upper lids, lashes, and brows were darkened with galena, a dark kohl-like paint. The galena was drawn into winged lines at the outside corner of each eye. The result was beautiful, enlarged, expressive eyes.

The mouth is another focal point of the face. My grandmother used to tell me that as long as you've got a smile on, you're fully dressed for any occasion. A smile may be a sign of shyness, friendship, or blissful happiness, but one thing is undeniable: a smile is a definite enhancement to any face.

Not all cultures agree, though, on what a smile should look like. In some parts of Central Africa and Sumatra, people file their teeth into sharp points to enhance their beauty. In Bali, by contrast, sharp teeth, even incisors, are associated with monsters, and the teeth are filed flat as a sign that someone is considered a full member of the society. In Senegal and Morocco, where shining white teeth are a much-desired beauty attribute, many women play tricks with contrast. Moroccan women chew on *souek*, a tree bark that darkens the gum slightly and makes the teeth seem brighter by comparison. In traditional Senegal, when women come of age, they undergo a gum-tattooing ritual. As with many coming-of-age ceremonies, there is a test of worthiness. The gum tattooing is quite painful and the young women must demonstrate their bravery by not crying out during the operation. Dr. Ndioro Ndiaye, a professor of dentistry at the University of Dakar, Senegal, who incidentally has tattooed gums herself, insists that the tattooing not only makes the teeth seem whiter, it also helps prevent gum diseases. In fact, this traditional method of dental hygiene is being looked at more closely and is enjoying a new popularity in modern Senegal. Tattooing has become a procedure that contemporary Senegalese women can have done, not in the dusty courtyard of a relative's home, but in the sterile environment of an up-to-date dentist's office.

Fresh breath is another universal beauty attribute. While the Masai's remedy of cow urine and ash may seem a bit drastic, the Native American use of sage and the traditional African American use of baking soda hit a bit closer to home. Once their teeth are cleaned, Indian women will chew fennel or anise seeds after a meal to freshen their breath. (Now you know what those baskets of seeds are as you leave your favorite Indian restaurant.) Breath fresheners like myrrh pastilles and cloves are also chewed to ensure that the breath is not offensive.

The women of Mali and several other West African nations use a chewing stick to clean their teeth and freshen their breath. The best ones are made from bitter, astringent woods. In Sandaga and Tilene markets in Dakar, Senegal, there are basketsful of them awaiting purchase. It is not uncommon to see a young woman in deep and rapt conversation with the vendor about the type and provenance of the wood. Some people are so particular about their chewing sticks that the Arabian poet Abu-I-Hawari

Wisati once wished in verse to be a chewing stick so that he could enjoy a young woman's mouth.

> *Good luck to the wood of the thorn tree that has the*
> *pleasure in me despite of serving as a tooth-stick*
> *in the sweet mouth of a pretty snub-nose girl!*

In many parts of the world, the toothpick, the baby sister of the tooth stick, is taken out of its shameful hiding place and proudly passed around after meals. After all, reason many, you must be well off to have meat on the table to stick in your teeth, so why not savor the cleaning up afterwards!

LET'S FACE IT

Eyes, mouth, nose, and complexion all come together in the part of you that is most identifiable as you. Your friends might not recognize your hands or your feet, but you certainly expect them to know you by your face.

The best way to start to find your beauty is from the inside out. Watch not only what you eat—don't neglect those vegetables and grains   but also what you think, the folks with whom you associate, your life, and your loves. Your face mirrors your entire life. If you're unhappy, you will never truly feel beautiful. Only when you have the right energies radiating outward can you begin with the externals.

FACIAL SCRUBS

Just as an artist begins with a clean canvas, so should you. First clean your face. To soap or not to soap then becomes the primary question, and women of the exotic world often disagree on this. When I was an adolescent suffering the torment of acne, a friend suggested that I try her remedy. It was as simple as going to the drugstore to purchase a bottle of tincture of green soap and a man's shaving brush.

Oily Skin Cleanser

Tincture of green soap (available at most pharmacies without a prescription)

Man's shaving brush

Pour a small amount of green soap onto the shaving brush. Wet your face with tepid water and then lather up with the brush as though you were going to shave. The brush is mildly abrasive and the soap fights infection. This should not be done on a daily basis, as too much stimulation will only increase the acne. Once or twice a week should be enough. Remember, this is for oily skin only. Those with dry, sensitive, or even combination/normal skin shouldn't try this.

Not sure if you have dry, oily, or combination/normal skin? You'll usually know if you have oily skin because suddenly in the middle of the afternoon you'll feel as though you've been freshly dipped in Crisco, or because you've had breakouts and blackheads all your life. Women with dry skin don't have these problems, but they're more sensitive to sunburn and windburn. Combination/normal skin has a bit of each, usually an oily zone around the forehead and nose. Each type has its pluses and minuses. Women with dry skin enjoy beautiful complexions, while women with oilier skin languish with pimples and bumps. We come into our own later, though, because oily skin does not age as rapidly. Many women of color have oily skin—one of the reasons that African American women's faces do not age at the same rate as those of their Anglo counterparts.

Women of color with dry skin can take solace in a traditional African American remedy—one that, like most, comes from the kitchen. This one calls for mayonnaise.

⚒

Martha's Mayonnaise Magic

1 tablespoon mayonnaise

When ready to wash your face, apply the mayonnaise in a thin sheet. Then massage lightly with your fingertips in upward motions until you have covered your entire face. Leave the mayonnaise on for a few minutes before rinsing off thoroughly with several rinses of clear, tepid water. The oil in the mayonnaise lightly moisturizes the skin.

Every now and then a good facial scrub is the perfect complexion cleanser. This idea is not new but harks back to the Egyptians. The following variation comes from a cousin of mine who lived in Egypt briefly.

⚒

Yvette's Almond Meal Scrub

1 tablespoon finely ground almond meal
(available at health-food stores)
1½ teaspoons fresh milk

Place the almond meal in the palm of your hand and add enough of the milk to make an abrasive paste. (You may need a bit more or a bit less; this will depend on the texture of the almond meal.) Apply the paste to your face with the fingertips and scrub lightly, using small circular movements of the fingertips. When finished with the entire face, rinse thoroughly with tepid water. Pat dry with a clean towel.

Almonds, though, are relatively expensive and so is almond meal. You can get similar results with an African American standby using cornmeal.

Grandma's And-You-Thought-Cornmeal-Was-Just-for-Cornbread Scrub

    1½ tablespoons yellow cornmeal
    2 tablespoons plain yogurt

Mix the cornmeal and yogurt together in the palm of your hand until it forms a grainy liquid. Apply the liquid to your face, massaging lightly with the balls of your fingers. Rinse well with tepid water and pat dry with a clean towel.

In the southwestern United States and Mexico, two Native American staples are avocados and corn. When they're not being eaten in a variety of delicious dishes, they sometimes find their way into the bathroom and bedroom, where they're used to create a gentle facial scrub that rids the skin of impurities and gives the complexion a healthy glow.

Corn Maiden Scrub

½ ripe avocado
2 teaspoons finely ground yellow cornmeal

In a small bowl, mix the ingredients thoroughly with a fork until you have a grainy paste. Wash your face thoroughly and then apply the avocado-cornmeal mixture. Gently rub the mixture over your face, paying special attention to trouble spots where you are prone to blackheads and blemishes. Rinse the mixture off with a flood of tepid water. Rinse at least ten times, as the cornmeal is stubborn and quite difficult to remove. Finish off the masque with a splash of cold water and pat the face dry with a clean towel.

Skin scrubs are good for an occasional pick-me-up for all but the most sensitive skin types. The following skin cleanser comes from my friend Khadijah, who has worked in herb stores and beauty parlors most of her adult life. She devised an inside-out cleansing system that cleanses the skin perfectly and leaves it ready for a facial masque.

Khadijah's Inside-Out Tea Party

It's really quite simple: infuse a double batch of herbs into a tea by allowing them to steep in hot water; drink some of the tea to clean out your system; and use the rest to steam your face. This way you're working on cleaning your body from the inside out. Khadijah uses chamomile, because she has dry skin and the steam softens it. Other herbs that can be used include lavender, a natural antibacterial and a soother; lemon balm, which is good for depression and nervous exhaustion; and mint, which is good for migraines.

3   cups water

1   stainless steel or ceramic pot

3   tablespoons of the dried herb to be used

1   tea infuser

1   mug or teacup for the tea

1   towel

Heat the water to almost boiling in a kettle. Place one tablespoon of the dried herb in the tea infuser. Place the tea infuser in a mug and add water until the mug is full. Allow the tea to infuse for ten minutes. While the tea is infusing, allow the remaining water to come to a full boil. Then, place the remaining two tablespoons of the herb in a bowl, pour the boiling water over it, and lean over the bowl, draping your head with a towel so that you are inhaling the vapors from the herb. Allow your face to absorb as much steam as possible, but be careful not to bend so close that you burn yourself. Remain as long as you can stand the heat or until the water cools. Then pat your face dry with a clean towel, sip the tea slowly, and don't go out into the cold for at least a half hour. You'll have a glow that will come from the inside out.

FACIAL MASQUES

Facial masques are used throughout the world. Burmese women rub on a gold paste made from the bark of the chenakat tree. The bark, which is ground into a fine powder before being applied, is said to "keep the skin tight." In parts of India, sandalwood powder is used as a facial masque, and everything from papaya to avocado is dabbed on the face in the New World. The earliest known facial masques go back to the Egyptians. One is still used today and is sitting in your refrigerator waiting for you to discover it.

Egyptian Egg Masque

1 egg

It's that simple. Separate the egg into two small bowls, taking care to keep the yolk from the white. (Save the yolk to enrich your next shampoo.) Then, after you have cleaned your face and perhaps steamed it with Khadijah's Inside-Out Tea Party, slather the egg white on your face. It's a bit slimy, but it will tighten up after a while. Leave the masque on your face for fifteen minutes or until it becomes dry and tight. Then rinse off with tepid water, pat dry with a clean towel, and feel revitalized.

When you're down in the dumps, it tends to show first in your complexion. A tried-and-true African American facial masque calls for brewer's yeast to brighten up the complexion. My friend Martha Mae from Chesapeake Bay, who's wise in the traditional ways of African Americans, swears by it.

Martha's Pick-Me-Up

> 1 tablespoon brewer's yeast
> Tepid water

Place the brewer's yeast in the palm of your hand and add enough tepid water to form a thin paste. Apply the paste all over the face and neck area. Allow it to dry and keep it on the face for about ten minutes. Remove it with a thorough rinse of tepid water and then pat the face dry with a clean towel.

The scent of sandalwood is enough to transport me back to a wonderful trip that I made to India several years ago. I recall the brilliant colors: shocking pinks, peacock turquoises, and deep, iridescent greens. I remember the particular, not unpleasant, smell of cow-dung cooking fires, the kind, welcoming ways of the people, the dazzling art and architecture of Rajasthan, and the willingness of the women to share their beauty secrets. One that I learned was for an instant sandalwood masque.

Instant India Facial Masque

> 1 tablespoon sandalwood powder (Indian women pulverize their own on a pumice stone, but it can be purchased from most health-food stores or herbalists)
> Warm water

Using that ever-present, ever-popular container that is the palm of your hand, place the sandalwood powder into your hand. Add water a few drops at a time until you have a paste. Apply the paste to your face and savor the sandalwood scent. Allow the masque to remain for ten minutes or until it has dried completely. Rinse with tepid water and then pat dry with a clean towel. You'll feel as fresh as if you'd journeyed to the Vale of Kashmir.

Caribbean women have a way with facials as well. The region's bounty of tropical fruits and vegetables gives them ample ingredients with which to work, and over the centuries they have devised wonderful ways of keeping their complexions fresh and clear in the Antillean sun. Papaya has been featured in many of them. It is particularly wonderful for oily skin. Papaya works well because the same enzymes that make it a natural meat tenderizer also help the skin to gently slough off dead cells and look clearer. I got this recipe from Dorotea.

Papaya Purifier

1 small ripe papaya (it must be fresh!)

Peel the papaya and place the pulp in the bowl of a blender or food processor. Pulse until you have a creamlike liquid. Apply the papaya cream to the face and leave it on for fifteen minutes. Rinse thoroughly with cool water, and see how your skin glows and feels refreshed.

Alternately, if you simply cannot pass up the taste of a fresh papaya and feel that it's too good to waste on your face, rub the inner side of the peeled papaya skin over your face. Because the small fibers on the inside of the skin are slightly abrasive, the inner skin will also work the papaya's magic on your complexion.

Another secret that I wormed out of Dorotea was her seasonal facial masque. At the change of every season, when almost all complexions get a bit muddy with the changes of weather, Dorotea would perk up her face with a five-day treatment with *barro*. *Barro* simply means clay in Spanish, but the *barro* that Dorotea was using was special. It was a red clay that was sold only by a neighborhood woman. I walked all over Old San Juan, checking out the neighborhood pharmacies, but I was unable to duplicate Dorotea's exact clay. Then, at Vineyard Sound Herbs, an herbalist's shop on Martha's Vineyard Island, last summer, I found a red clay that just does the job. You can find red facial clay at your local herbalist or order it from Vineyard Sound Herbs (see mail-order sources in appendix A).

Dorotea's Five-Day Seasonal Pick-Me-Up

2 ounces powdered red facial clay

Every evening for five days, prepare the following masque for your face. Place one tablespoon of the red clay in the palm of your hand and mix it with enough water to make a thin paste. Apply the paste to your face, avoiding the eye area, and to your neck. Leave the masque on for ten minutes or until it has thoroughly dried. Then rinse it off with tepid water and pat the face dry with a clean towel.

You'll notice that pimples may appear after the first few days. Don't despair. That's only the skin ridding itself of its impurities. Toward the end of the five-day period, the skin will clear up and exude radiant health. Remember, though, this is a treatment for oily skins, and one that should only be used seasonally. Single applications of the masque may be used occasionally during the interim period.

We can also head back to the kitchen and concoct various masques for our faces from familiar ingredients. My mother passed the following recipe along to me.

Mama's Oatmeal Masque

2 tablespoons oatmeal	1 egg white
2 teaspoons wildflower honey	

Mix the ingredients together in a small bowl until they form a thick paste. Slather the paste onto clean skin and allow it to remain for fifteen minutes. Rinse the paste off thoroughly with tepid water. Finish with a splash of cool water and pat dry. The oatmeal is good for oily skin, as it will help remove the excess oil.

In Malaysia, renowned beauties have relied for centuries on small white pellets called *bedak sejok.* These pellets are prepared from fermented rice, mixed with water, and used as a toning masque to promote smooth, clear skin. *Bedak sejok* is thought to have been one of the primary beauty secrets of the legendary Malaysian beauty Lena Bobo.

I took down the recipe for the preparation of *bedak sejok* one afternoon while sitting with some artisans in a batik factory in Penang, Malaysia. The hand-printed cloth that I bought from them in gratitude for the company and the recipe is beautiful, but one day it will be no more. Lena Bobo's beauty secret lasts forever. If you've got time and lots of patience, you can prepare your own. (The process takes five months.) If not, you can salute the diligence and the inventiveness of exotic women of color around the world who spend time preparing unguents and potions to enhance their beauty. Here is the recipe.

Bedak Sejok

1 large, clean, widemouthed jar or crock
Unprocessed white rice
Water
1 small, clean funnel
1 square yard clean white muslin

Place the rice and water into the jar. The proportions should be two-thirds rice to one-third water; the amounts will depend on the size of the jar. Place the jar in a cool place and allow the rice to soak. Change the water on the rice every two days, maintaining the proportions of one-third water to two-thirds rice. Be sure to leave enough room in the jar or crock to allow the rice to expand. Let the rice ferment. This process will take about five months.

When the rice is soft and liquid, pour the liquid into the funnel. Use the tube of the funnel to dot pea-sized balls of the fermented rice onto the clean white muslin. Place the cloth on a tray and allow the small balls to harden in the sun. You may want to place them in a two-hundred-degree oven overnight to hasten this process, but at this point, what's a few more days. When the *bedak sejok* is ready, store it in a jar that can be tightly closed.

When ready to use as a masque, take two of the small balls in the palm of your hand and add enough water to transform them into a white paste that's fairly liquid. Apply the paste to your face and allow it to remain for fifteen to twenty minutes. Rinse off with warm water and then pat dry with a clean towel. If you've taken five months to prepare this, you'll feel at one with the Malaysian women and as refreshed and lovely as Lena Bobo herself.

If you have dry skin, you need not despair; the world of exotic women of color offers facial masques for you as well. When I was working as a travel writer, I covered southern Asia for *Travel Weekly,* a newspaper for travel agents. At that time, I had many friends at the Indian tourist office in New York City. One of them not only gave me a wealth of information on that land of mysteries; she also gave me this recipe for an excellent skin masque for dry or normal skin.

Crème Indienne

> 1 tablespoon heavy cream
> ½ lime

Place the heavy cream in a small bowl. Squeeze the lime into the bowl. The lime juice will "turn" the cream slightly, but not to worry. Slather the mixture on your face. Leave it on for about twenty minutes, then rinse off with warm water. You'll find that the cream is moisturizing and the bit of lime juice is astringent and adds a slight tingle.

My Mexicana friend Beatriz is a never-ending source of information on the traditional beauty secrets of Mexico. One day, as we were wandering through Libertad market in Guadalajara, she told me this one, which uses parsley.

------------------------------------ ❦ ------------------------------------

Beatriz's Mexican Moisturizing Masque

1 tablespoon minced parsley

1 tablespoon honey

1 tablespoon milk

Place all the ingredients in a small bowl and blend them into a thin paste. Apply the paste to the face and allow it to remain for twenty minutes. Then rinse off with warm water. Add a splash of cold water to refresh, and pat dry with a clean towel.

One of the joys of teaching for me is that over the years I have had students from many nations in my classroom. In the course of a semester we work on many different assignments, some of them involving the family traditions of their various lands. One day, while doing just such an exercise, a young woman from Colombia came up with this moisturizing masque that was traditional in her family. It's perfect for all skin types, including dry skin.

------------------------------------ ❦ ------------------------------------

Isabel's Moisturizing Masque

1 tablespoon fresh honey

Simply moisten the face slightly with warm water, then dab the honey all over. Leave the honey on for half an hour. It will become slightly tacky and sticky by then. Rinse well and finish off with a splash of cold water and a pat with a clean towel.

Honey has been used in facial treatments for centuries. Just about every culture has a honey masque. They range from the simple, like Isabel's, to the complex, which require multiple ingredients. Try adding ingredients to the honey for your own personalized masque. In Mexico, they add one tablespoon of light cream to the tablespoon of honey for a cream-and-honey complexion. My grandmother used to add a few drops of lavender water to her tablespoon of honey for a facial masque. The possibilities are limited only by your inventiveness.

Like honey, the avocado turns up in a variety of facial treatments in the New World where it originated. From peel to pit, this wonderful fruit is the queen of the beauty table.

While roaming in the Mercado Modelo in Santo Domingo, among the rocking chairs and the *pan de casave,* I found a woman at the door with a basketful of perfectly ripe avocados. She urged me to purchase not one, but two, luring me with the thought that even if I couldn't eat them both, I could use one of them for a facial masque.

Mercado Masque

1 small ripe avocado

Peel the avocado, remove the pit, and mash the pulp into a paste with a fork. You can also do this, if you're not in a hotel room as I was, with a blender. Simply peel the avocado, pit it, and pop it into the blender. Blend at low speed until it becomes a paste. Apply the avocado cream to the face and leave the masque on for twenty minutes. Then rinse thoroughly with warm water and tone with a splash of cold water before you pat dry with a clean towel.

The avocado-paste idea that the Dominicana had given me is actually not a new one; it goes back as far as pre-Colombian America. The Incas simply applied avocado paste to the skin and massaged it in. After a while, they removed the residue. This masque is particularly good for those in need of a moisturizer, as the avocado oil remains on for a time and is absorbed by the skin.

Beatriz would have to turn in her title as beauty whiz if she didn't have at least one recipe for an avocado masque. She has provided me with one of the best masques of all. It combines honey and cream with the avocado for a masque that is moisturizing and delicious.

Beatriz's Beautifier

½ ripe avocado   ¼ cup heavy cream
1 tablespoon honey

Place all the ingredients in a bowl and blend at low speed until you have a thin paste. Alternately, you can mash the avocado with a fork and gradually add the honey and cream until you have a thin paste. Whatever method, when you have the paste, lather it onto your face and neck. Relax and try not to lick your face for twenty to thirty minutes. Then remove the masque with several rinses of tepid water and finish up with a toning splash of cold water. Pat dry with a clean towel, and enjoy your fresh glow.

Virtually all parts of the avocado can be used in various beauty treatments. Nothing has to go to waste. Take the peels and rub the interior on your face. The slightly grainy texture of the inside of the avocado peel is exfoliating, and the peel itself is rich with avocado oil. The combination is great for those with problem skin. Also, don't forget to eat avocados; they're rich in vitamins A, C, and E, iron, potassium, niacin, and protein. That helps build beauty from the inside out.

Beatriz not only won the most-avocado-uses title with her avocado masque; she topped herself with a use for the avocado that I had never heard of and a tale that mystified and fascinated me. I call it the Tale of the Pit.

The Tale of the Pit

The avocado pit is a perfect applicator. It fits well into the palm of your hand and can be rolled easily over the face to help any cream spread evenly. The action of the pit rolling over the face is both soothing and exercising. Place the pit in your right hand to apply creams and exercise the left side of your face, and vice versa. You'll be fascinated by the soothing feel.

You do not have to do anything special to the pit itself. Simply remove it from the avocado and wipe it off. You'll have the extra benefit of a bit of the avocado oil that it generates as well.

TONERS

The skin cleansed and refreshed, the time has come to tone. This is done most simply by applying a slightly astringent toner to the face to complete the process. There are various types of skin fresheners, but one of my favorites is still one that good old Mom recommended years ago.

Mom's Skin Toner

1 tablespoon cider vinegar

1 cup mineral water

Mix the cider vinegar and the mineral water together and place them in a bottle that can be tightly sealed. You may wish to keep this mixture in the refrigerator. The extra chill will make it more refreshing.

I love lemons in everything and was delighted when some friends suggested that I should stop running all over Dakar, Senegal, trying to find cider vinegar and simply use the variation on this recipe that they did. It called for lemon juice.

Nicole's Lemon Lotion

2   lemons
1½ cups cold mineral water

Squeeze the lemons and strain the juice into a small bottle. Add the mineral water. Use as an astringent toner after any of the facial masques.

Cucumbers also make a wonderful skin toner. They have slight bleaching properties that make them perfect for clearing up muddied complexions. My new Martiniquaise friend, Madame Renée, told me how generations of women have prepared cucumber milk.

Lait de Concombre

1 fresh cucumber

You really need a farmer's-market cucumber for this. Simply slice off the stem end of the cucumber. Then, picking up the slice by the stem, slowly rub the slice over the cut made in the cucumber. After you have rubbed the two cut surfaces of the cucumber together for a few minutes, a pale green milklike liquid will begin to form. That's the cucumber milk. Dab it onto your face, and then go on and eat your salad complete with the rest of the cucumber.

Can't find farmer's-market cucumbers? Try this freshener that's almost a masque.

Cucumber Fresh-Up

1 small cucumber   1 egg white

Peel the cucumber and seed it by cutting it in half lengthwise and scooping out the tiny seeds with a spoon. Place it in the bowl of a blender and pulse until it is a watery paste. In a separate bowl, beat the egg white into a froth and then fold the cucumber mixture into the egg white. Apply the mixture, which will be drippy, to the skin and allow it to remain for ten to fifteen minutes. Then rinse off with a flood of cool water and towel dry.

A smooth, lustrous complexion is a beauty plus almost anywhere in the world, but our Asian sisters seem to place particular emphasis on the pearly smoothness of their skin. In fact, at Chinese herbalists' shops in Taiwan, Hong Kong, and Singapore, in among the herbs and pickled snakes on the display counters, there are always champagne glasses full of tiny seed pearls. These pearls are pulverized, mixed with water or another liquid, and taken internally to promote skin as soft, smooth, and lustrous as a pearl. This case of sympathetic cosmetology has Egyptian parallels. Cleopatra is said to have drunk wine with a pearl dissolved in it. There are many others, all wonderful examples of the inventiveness of women of color. Drinking liquefied pearls is an expensive beauty treatment; others, though, are not as hard on the pocketbook.

The Egyptian Ebers Papyrus prescribed a mixture of cake meal and well water for a smooth complexion and suggested that women anoint their faces with it daily after washing. Vietnamese women have found a new solution for the thorny problem of what to do with all those artichoke leaves. They brew the leaves into an infusion that is dabbed on skin flare-ups to clear them up.

FRECKLE FADERS, COMPLEXION ENHANCERS, AND SKIN PROBLEMS

Several treatises would be needed to explain the nuances of the minefield known as color in the world of women of darker hue. European ideals of beauty have so traumatized many that all manners of creams, treatments, and potions have been evolved to bleach and fade away natural pigmentation. In Senegal, where during the 1970s this need to have light skin reached epic proportions, women came up with a noxious mixture of Clorox, French shampoo, and other ingredients that was called *xessel*. The substance was so caustic that women had to hop around after applying it; it burned that much.

The end result of this sorrowful testimonial to a lesser-known, yet psychically harmful, consequence of colonialism was a skin that was no longer the deep, rich, eggplant-hued black of many of the country's belles, but rather a raw, reddish burnt umber. *Xessel* was not the only product used. Those with vast amounts of money would journey abroad to have injections of a substance originally used in leather tanning, which would leave them with similar raw, reddish complexions. All of this pain and spiritual suffering in the quest for a European ideal of beauty. Happily, today all skin-bleaching products are outlawed in Senegal. They also now have their own traditional beauty pageant celebrating the aesthetic that is theirs. The winners are often gap-toothed (a gap between the two front teeth is a sign of great beauty), lush of figure (this is the country of the *diryanke* or large-figured courtesan), and deep rich purply black of skin.

The Senegalese experience notwithstanding, women of African descent do sometimes have uneven complexions and discolored spots on their faces and bodies. Mild creams with bleaching properties have also traditionally been used to even up these discolorations.

In the Dominican Republic, women use two methods to clear them up. They mix Palmer's ointment, an over-the-counter patent medicine, and Vaseline together. The mixture is then applied to blemishes and pimples in the evening and left on overnight. Even though the Vaseline attenuates the strength of the Palmer's ointment a bit, it is a strong mixture that reacts to sunlight.

Legend has it that Josephine Baker brightened and cleared her complexion by rubbing herself all over with fresh lemons. Whether or not this is true, and much that is recounted about La Baker is most emphatically not true, it is undeniable that the lemon has good bleaching properties. Rub half a lemon over your dark spots or rough elbows for a few weeks and watch them slowly fade to their original hue.

The ancient Chinese believed that sorrel juice could remove freckles. I'm never going to have freckles in this lifetime, but if you do, you might want to purchase a bunch of fresh sorrel (the green leafy kind, not the pods used to brew the West Indian drink, which are red and related to the hibiscus plant).

---- ✄ ----

Chinese Freckle Fader

1 bunch fresh sorrel leaves	Surgical gauze

Wash the sorrel thoroughly. Then prepare a chiffonade by rolling the leaves together and slicing them crosswise into thin strips. Prepare a compress by placing the sorrel strips between several sheets of gauze about four inches long by three inches wide. Place the compress over the freckles to be faded and allow it to remain for fifteen minutes. The sorrel compress will begin to fade the freckles. Continue to apply the compresses every two or three days until the freckles fade. Don't expect instant miracles; remember, Mother Nature works slowly. If you get impatient with the time that it's taking, you can always use the remaining sorrel for a wonderful French *soupe à l'oseille.*

Buttermilk, one of the favorite beverages of the American South, is a perfect bleach for freckles or spots on delicate skins. If you really want to pamper yourself, try this one.

---- ✄ ----

Buttermilk Bliss

½ cup fresh buttermilk	Surgical gauze

Form the gauze into compresses by cutting it into sections and folding it into pieces about four inches long by three inches wide and several layers thick. Saturate the gauze compresses with the buttermilk. Apply the compresses to your blemishes. Leave them on for thirty minutes or so—longer if you fall asleep. When through, rinse thoroughly with cool water. Slowly, but surely, with this treatment, the dark spots will begin to fade away.

For slightly faster results, follow in Josephine Baker's footsteps and turn to lemons.

Baker's Bleach

½ cup freshly squeezed lemon juice
Surgical gauze

Prepare two gauze compresses and saturate them with the lemon juice. Apply the compresses to your dark or discolored areas and allow them to remain for twenty minutes or so. Then relax, knowing that Mother Nature is at work. If you're using lemon juice as a bleaching agent, be sure to avoid the sun after application, as the lemon may react to the sun's rays and cause unsightly dark spots.

Those of you with more sensitive skin might want to avoid the lemon and think of using cucumber pulp on the compresses instead. You can mix the cucumber pulp with buttermilk. It will take a bit longer, but your delicate complexion will thank you.

A final hint about breakouts from the people of the Winnebago nation. They used oil collected from boiling the leaves of the wild bergamot plant to dry up pimples. You can get similar benefits by simply dabbing the offending pimple with a tiny bit of essential oil of bergamot diluted with sweet almond oil or witch hazel.

THE EYES HAVE IT

Eyes are one of the most expressive parts of your body. In countries where women are veiled and only their eyes are visible, they use their eyes to convey all human emotions. Try it yourself. Drape an opaque scarf around your head and lower face. Cover all but your eyes. Now see how they begin to take over. See how expressive they can be. Practice using them: question, smile, flirt, dazzle. Learn to use your eyes to your best advantage. It goes without saying that you should take care of your eyes—they are not only the mirrors of the soul, but also the mirrors of health. Regular ophthalmological checkups will not only tell you about the health of your eyes; they will reveal much about your general health as well. Your ophthalmologist can tell whether other organs are in good condition by looking into your eyes. As far back as the ancient Egyptians, doctors were aware of the connection between eye health and general health. They prescribed calves' liver for eye ailments. Eye makeups were used to protect the eyes from the hot desert sun. Salves were also prescribed, many of which contained collyrium mixed with various other ingredients, as the doctors came up with treatments for everything from bleary eyes to cataracts.

You must not only take medical care of your eyes; you must also treat them kindly. Tired, red, puffy eyes show the world that you've been burning the candle at both ends a bit too much. And while it may make a lovely light, it doesn't make for beautiful eyes.

The following recipes will soothe eyes fatigued from too many hours at the computer or too many hours spent in smoky or pollen-filled rooms and polluted city streets.

Theodora's Eye Magic

White potatoes are native to the New World and not frequently found in most West African markets. My friend Theodora has lived around the world, however, and somewhere along the way she came up with this recipe for eyes that are puffy or just in need of a little rest.

Surgical gauze	1 medium-sized white potato

Form the gauze into two compresses by cutting several pieces about four inches long by three inches wide. Peel and grate the potato, and place the potato pulp in the compresses. Apply the compresses to your closed eyes for thirty minutes or more. Relax and banish all thoughts of business, beaux, and other woes—just relax. When you're through, dab some cool water on your face and voilà, your eyes have been soothed and you'll feel revitalized and renewed.

I am a tea bag collector. My kitchen counter is frequently dotted with tea bags that I've used once but that are too good to throw away—after all, there's still some tea in there to be used. I finally took a hint from Martha, my ever-practical friend, who is a weaver and a dyer. She employs used tea bags to soothe her tired eyes in the African American tradition of waste not, want not.

꒜

Bag It Martha's Way

2 used tea bags

I like to use herbal tea bags like lavender or chamomile.

Simply apply the cooled tea bags to your eyes. If the tea bags have dried out, dampen them with a bit of lukewarm water. Sit back and allow them to soothe you for about fifteen minutes. There will be enough residual herbal essence in the tea bags to refresh you, and it gives you something to do with all those used tea bags.

Eyes brightened, what about their setting? Long, luxuriant eyelashes are a wonderful thing. Unfortunately, we are not all born with them. I learned this trick while living in a dormitory in Nancy, France, where I was astonished to see a fellow student retire to the communal bathroom each evening with a small bottle of castor oil and a mascara brush. Mystified, I watched and watched until finally curiosity got the best of me and I had to ask. The explanation was simple: she was brushing the castor oil through her eyelashes to make them grow. It doesn't happen overnight, but if you're as diligent as my friend was, you will be rewarded. Years later, while reading a translation of the Ebers Papyrus, I was amazed to find that the ancient Egyptians had recommended using castor oil for hair growth as well.

In Mexico, one summer, I learned to curl my eyelashes without the aid of one of those complicated-looking pieces of equipment made for that task. My friend Beatriz simply used a teaspoon. You take the edge of a teaspoon, holding it so that the bowl of the spoon faces out, and curl the lashes by holding them in the fingers of one hand and running the spoon edge over the lashes.

Eye-black is popular in much of the Arab world. It goes under the names kohl, *surmane, kajal,* and *tutia* and is one of the more controversial of the world's cosmetics. One of the reasons for the controversy seems to be that there are many different recipes for making kohl. Traditional kohl is prepared from antimony and was used as far back as the ancient Egyptians, who believed that it protected their eyes from the hot sun. Many of the kohls that are for sale today, even in the traditional markets of Morocco and Tunisia, are no more than colored chemical powders. While antimony was originally thought to be protective, many now feel that it is harmful. Others—many kohl-wearing women among them—praise kohl because they feel it shields the eyes from impurities, protects them from common eye diseases, and guards against the evil eye, in addition to giving the wearer a smoky, sultry look. Kohl has been around for thousands of years and is more than likely here to stay. In Egypt and throughout the Middle East and North Africa, in India and in many parts of the world where Islam has spread, kohl is a way of life.

In ancient Egypt, different types of eye makeup were used at different times of the year, but no matter what the season, walking about without made-up eyes was inconceivable. Wearing eye makeup cut across class and gender boundaries, because the use was more protective (from the sun's rays) than simply cosmetic.

In the West, kohl had a vogue in the late nineteenth and early twentieth centuries, thanks to such famous users as Sarah Bernhardt and Theda Bara. It took the 1960s by storm when many looked to alternative makeup methods. Today, a number of companies manufacture eye pencils that purport to be kohl, but you should be aware that not all these products have the properties of traditionally prepared kohls. I'm a traditionalist and feel that if you're going to use kohl, there's nothing like the real thing. I even find that the kohl I can buy in the marketplace in Morocco is easier on my eyes than many of the pencils that I buy. If you too would like to try real kohl, find a reputable dealer who is selling the real thing, not an adulterated cosmetic. Head to an herbalist or to the Arab or Indian section of your town. You can also order kohl from the sources listed in the mail-order section. Then, all you need is patience and a steady hand.

Fatima, my Moroccan friend who first initiated me into the mysteries of kohl, gave me interesting advice for kohl use. First, if buying your own kohl in the market in Morocco, purchase it only from the little old ladies. They grind their own, and what's most important, they use their own. The kohl is likely to be purer. Fatima also told me to avoid the so-called colored kohls— they're only dyes that may or may not be pure. Finally, she told me that kohl has almost religious significance in Morocco. Some people even feel that the black stone from which it is ground represents the black stone of the Holy Kaaba at Mecca, one of the holiest points in Islam. She went on to tell me that the best kohls have a grain of pepper ground into them. This helps the eye to tear and rid itself of any impurities. Fatima was such an expert on kohl and its use that she had wormed a recipe for making it out of one of her little old ladies in the market. The recipe that follows is for your reading pleasure only. *Do not* attempt to make your own kohl.

To Make Kohl

Take a lemon, cut it in half, and remove the insides from one of the halves. Fill the lemon half with plumbago and burnt copper. Place the lemon half on a flame and allow it to burn until the entire lemon and contents are carbonized. Place the carbonized lemon in a mortar with a pinch of coral, a dash of ambergris, a small seed pearl or two, some sandalwood, and a part of the body of a chameleon and the wing of a bat. Moisten the whole with rose water while hot.

I suspect the little old lady was pulling Fatima's leg with this recipe. She wasn't about to give away the secret of her livelihood.

On the day that Fatima took me through the weekly market in Agadir, we purchased some kohl from an old woman. It was sold, in true Moroccan fashion, in recycled serum containers. We then went on to buy a kohl applicator and a kohl box. The applicator is simply a short smooth stick that has been whittled down to a point at one end. The box is a cylinder made from turned wood and brightly decorated with hand-painted pink flowers. Wealthier women use kohl applicators of ivory and have kohl boxes of precious metals encrusted with jewels. Beyond their exteriors, though, all kohl boxes are the same. They're essentially long, narrow compartments in which the powdered kohl is stored.

Fatima demonstrated how to wet the stick, then twirl it around in the container until it is covered with just enough kohl. Then she showed me how to very carefully place the kohl stick on the ridge of my lower eyelid with the pointy end facing the inside corner of my eye, how to twist the stick slightly to loosen the kohl from the stick, and how to shut my eyes and draw the kohl stick slowly out from between my closed lids, leaving a fine line of smudgy kohl on my upper and lower inner eyelids. My application wasn't perfect the first time, but gradually I got the hang of it. I found that the kohl gave me a smoky, smudged, natural look that I can never quite manage to achieve with pencils. I also like the thought that in using traditional kohl, I inherit millennia of tradition.

TEETH

You can have the most sparkling eyes in the world and a smooth, poreless complexion, but no one will notice those assets if your mouth opens to reveal broken or decaying teeth. The world does not agree on an aesthetic for teeth—in some cultures, teeth are blackened; in others, they're filed down; and in still others, they're brushed to a pearly white—but you're probably happiest with white teeth and a fresh mouth.

Sage, the same herb that's in your kitchen cabinet and frequently in the dressing of your Thanksgiving turkey, has been used as a tooth freshener by both Native American peoples and Bedouin Arabs.

Bedouin Tooth Freshener

2 tablespoons ground dried sage

Wet your toothbrush and dip it into the sage, then brush your teeth as usual. You'll find that your teeth will feel clean and refreshed and so will your breath.

If you can get fresh sage leaves from your greengrocer or supermarket, you can simply rub a few of them over your teeth to clean your teeth in the true traditional Bedouin manner.

Myrrh is a substance that has been used medicinally for a long time. (Remember, it was one of the three kings' gifts to the infant Jesus in the Christian Bible?) It is excellent for the teeth because it is a mild disinfectant and a local stimulant to the mucous membranes. In many Arab countries, myrrh pastilles are chewed as breath fresheners. Aisha, a friend from Egypt with a dazzling smile, came up with this recipe, which blends the myrrh of Egypt with baking soda from the Western world.

Aisha's Tooth Freshener

2 tablespoons powdered myrrh
¼ pound baking soda

In a small bowl, combine the powdered myrrh and baking soda and mix thoroughly. Then place the mixture in a container that can be tightly sealed. Wet the toothbrush and dip it into the mixture. Brush as usual. Voilà. This will freshen your teeth and breath, and the mixture will keep in the tightly sealed container for quite a while.

In parts of India, a tooth cleanser called *manjum* is prepared from tobacco ash, black pepper, and salt. If you're feeling truly experimental, it is something that's easy enough to concoct from readily available ingredients. Experiment to get the proportions that work for you.

Many Africans brought their oral hygiene habits with them from Africa to the southern United States. Chewing sticks (and their Western cousins, toothpicks) have endured as popular methods of keeping teeth clean and fresh. Traditional tooth cleaners include charcoal and, turning once again to the kitchen, baking soda. This was long before the American Dental Association came out with its recommendations and long before Arm and Hammer went into the toothpaste business.

Baking Soda Tooth Powder

1 small box baking soda

Simply take a bit of baking soda in the palm of your hand, wet your toothbrush, and dip it into the baking soda. Brush as usual. The baking soda is slightly abrasive and will leave your mouth feeling superclean and refreshed. Some folks think that the baking soda has an unpleasant taste; I don't.

In Morocco, when Fatima was through regaling me with tales of kohl, she turned to other topics. As we walked through the tented rows of the market in Agadir, she pointed out little packets that seemed to be bunches of bark. She explained that the bark was *souek* and that it was chewed as a tooth cleanser. It not only cleans the teeth but also slightly darkens the gums, making the teeth seem whiter in comparison. I told Fatima that the same trick is used in Senegal and Mali by women who have their gums tattooed a pinkish blue hue.

Clean teeth are only part of a beautiful smile. If your breath could kill a cow, no one's going to get close enough to admire your pearly whites. Breath fresheners are hallmarks of true beauties in the world of exotic women of color.

In the southwestern United States, *yerba santa* was widely used as a breath freshener by Native American peoples. The leaves of the plant were dried in small balls, which were popped into the mouth and chewed. The leaves have a slightly astringent taste, but after a glass of water, the mouth is refreshed.

The ancient Assyrians chewed fenugreek to banish bad breath. Cardamom and fennel are chewed in India for the same reason. Other breath fresheners range from parsley, which will even neutralize garlic mouth, to cloves, which were used as breath fresheners as far back as the third century B.C.

People also chew on aromatic gums and resins like copal and frankincense. Copal is a natural resin that has been burned as a religious incense by the Aztecs and their descendants for centuries. It has a curious taste, but one that is strangely refreshing.

Occasionally, all of us can be plagued by toothaches, but they can be temporarily conquered with a clove or two. This will work only briefly, but it makes the drive to the dentist easier.

Mommy and Daddy's Clove Cure

3–5 dried whole cloves or a drop or two of oil of cloves

Apply the fresh clove to the tooth that is hurting and bite down. The oil from the dried clove will soothe the tooth until you get to the dentist.

Alternately, you can dip a bit of cotton into oil of cloves and place the cotton on the sore tooth.

MAKEUP AND OTHER FINISHING TOUCHES

Aside from the heavy white makeup bases of Japan and China, makeup bases are not traditionally used by women of color. There's no need to add color to our faces. The touches that finish off a look, then, have more to do with decorating the lips and adding a bit of extra color to the cheeks.

In Trinidad, my friend Marlene was out driving with me one day when suddenly she stopped and pointed out a bush growing by the roadside. "Those are *roucou* berries," she explained, indicating a bush covered with small red berries. "They were originally used by the native peoples to decorate their bodies and incidentally to repel insects." It was only later that I discovered that *roucou* berries are also known as *achiote* or annatto (*Bixa orellana*) and that the plant is sometimes called the lipstick bush. The seeds are most often used today as a natural food coloring, giving much of the food of the Spanish Caribbean its distinctive reddish orange hue. However, if you're adventurous and looking for a new reddish orange color to add blush to your lips and cheeks, try this trick that I learned from María Elena, a Puerto Rican friend.

Carib Cheek Stain

Achiote (available in health-food stores or in supermarkets in Hispanic areas)

Rose water

Take four or five pieces of *achiote* and add them to a tablespoon of rose water. Allow the rose water to absorb the color of the *achiote*. When you have the desired color, take a cotton ball and apply the colored rose water as a cheek or lip stain. Be careful, though: while this color is not permanent, you might have to live with a mistake a little longer than you want.

Back in Morocco with Fatima, I found yet another beauty bonus, small clay pots of a reddish stain known as *akkar*. These small pots are found in markets and stalls all over the country. They are traditionally a part of the cosmetic arsenal of Berber women, who apply a clownlike blob on each cheek. It's easily transformed into a more contemporary cheek and lip stain by simply wetting a finger, dipping it in, and applying the *akkar* to the desired area.

In Haiti, where the women are ever ingenious, someone discovered years ago that pulverized brick made an excellent blusher for those who could not afford more traditional makeup. In India, where women prefer an amber glow to their skins, a finely pulverized powder of turmeric, which is yellow to orange, is used instead of the red-to-pink spectrum more popular in the West.

In many nations, whether it is a rosy glow or an amber hue, a final dusting of powder is what completes a woman's toilette. In Japan, geisha use a liberal dusting of rice powder to set their chalk-white makeup and add to their pallor. In old Cuba, where lighter-skinned women wanted to maintain their pallid complexions, they pulverized eggshells to make a powder called *cascarilla*. Try your own.

Cascarilla de Vieja Cuba

Several dozen clean, dried white eggshells

Simply retain the shells of white eggs after you have used them. Rinse them out and place them in the sun to dry out. When you have several dozen, you can proceed with the *cascarilla*. Place the eggshells in a paper bag and pulverize them with a rolling pin by rolling the pin over the paper bag several times. You can check on the shells as you roll. You'll know when they begin to look fine enough to go through a sieve. When they are completely pulverized, sieve them through a fine sieve until you have a fine powder. Place the powder in a container that can be tightly closed. That's the *cascarilla*. Use it when you want a chalk-white sophisticated pallor.

Not to be outdone, brown-skinned women developed their own look. They used *canela,* cinnamon. Not only was it cheaper than many face powders, it was readily available in the kitchens where many of the dark-skinned women worked, and it gave the complexion a wonderful matte look. Just a pat or two did the trick. The cinnamon had the added benefit of a spicy fragrance.

Clean face, eyes agleam with life, fresh mouth, and all of your finishing touches in place, all you need is a smile to meet anything that the world can offer. After all, you've put your best face forward.

⚘

Chapter 5

YOUR BODY

The Skin You're In

Some like 'em built for comfort;
Some like 'em built for speed.
TRADITIONAL BLUES

The woman I love is fat
Chocolate to the bone.
Every time she shakes,
Some skinny woman loses her home.
TRADITIONAL BLUES

FROM DIMINUTIVE CHINESE grandmothers who look as though they might blow away in a strong wind to stolid and solid matriarchs from Tonga who look as sturdy and as venerable as redwoods, we come not only in all colors, but in all sizes and shapes. Many of us, though, particularly those of us living in the United States, look in the mirror and see someone who is too short, too fat, too skinny, or too something else.

Wherever we live, we could all take a lesson from the majestic Senegalese courtesans known as *diryankes,* whose motto is: I've got a belly; I've got a butt; watch me strut! Just watching a *diryanke* strut her stuff on a narrow Dakar street is a lesson in feeling good about yourself, whatever your size. Her multicolored boubou billowing around her more-than-ample form in the Cap Vert breeze makes her look like a fantasy ship under full sail. She has a presence, a dignity, and a style that no waiflike model can ever hope for.

Think of that the next time you stare into the mirror and bemoan the effects of those french fries you shouldn't have eaten! Think, also, that in most of the world, where food is still savored and not suspect, a well-endowed form is a sign of prosperity. The argument, though, is not about being too fat or too skinny or even just right. In fact, there's really no argument. You can be fat or thin, have tattoos or be design-free, be tall or short, long-waisted, short-waisted, or no-waisted. The point is to have a healthy, well-groomed body with glowing skin, and to be comfortable with it. The French have an expression, *"être bien dans sa peau"* (to feel good in one's skin), to describe the inner confidence that results in an outwardly beautiful body.

Whether the ideal of beauty is callipygian or reed thin, all the world's cultures delight in a beautiful body. Over the centuries, they have developed all manner of beauty rituals to cleanse, enhance, and adorn the body.

Bathing was undoubtedly the first way that people began to respond to caring for the body. As a charter member of Bathers Anonymous, I think it's shameful that there's no monument to the first bather. In my mind I salute her, for it was certainly a woman, one who could not resist the lure of a shallow stream of fresh water in the middle of a sylvan grove or an unexpected waterfall tumbling down into a pool of limpid purity. She saw and could not help but dip in, first, a tentative toe and slowly, gradually, her whole body. Settling in, she discovered the calming, cleansing pleasures of the bath.

Although the Yoruba have no *orișa* of bathing, ritual baths are given for various *orișa,* and Oșun, the riverine goddess of coquetry, beauty, and wealth, is very much associated with bathing. It is not for naught that early civilizations developed at the edges of rivers; perhaps people recognized Oșun's civilizing qualities? Certainly they recognized the purifying, calming, life-giving force of water. We don't think about it much today, yet the primeval sacredness of water is still inherent in many of the world's religions, from the Christian baptism, to the burning ghats of Varanasi in India, the pre-prayer ablutions of Islam, and the purifying baths of Yoruba initiation.

By the time that we arrive at recorded history, folks have caught on to the notion of bathing with a vengeance. A bath found at Mohenjo-Daro in Pakistan is estimated to be some six thousand years old; another at Babylon is five thousand years old. By 3000 B.C., the Egyptians were even showering. Even though early Egyptian palaces often contained bathrooms, many people still bathed in the rivers. Bathrooms with ceramic pipes existed in Minoan Crete, and ancient India and Syria both had sophisticated bathing facilities with plumbing that works even today.

Bathing gradually went beyond the ritual to the sensory and was done just for the pleasure of it. Soaps, body scrubs, unguents, oils, and perfumes all developed out of the desire to enhance the bathing experience and more thoroughly purify, cleanse, and beautify the body.

Bathing draws with it a host of creamy unguents and ointments, of fragrant bubbles and oils and mousses, of soothing lotions and smoothers, abrasive mitts, pumices, and refreshing milk baths and coolers. All work to create and maintain the body beautiful. Once out of the bath, there are soothing massage oils and fragrant perfumes to entice, entrance, or just enjoy. Think of the sensuous massages prescribed by the *Kama Sutra* or the tender maternal massages that West African mothers give their infants.

Taking care of your body, inside and out, is your duty. You've only got one, and the replacement parts are few, far between, and usually made of plastic. Work with what you've got, enhance it, and embellish it. Caring for your body is enjoyable. Of all beauty rituals, it is perhaps the one that most combines the meditative and the worldly, the secular and the spiritual. It's one of the few totally sybaritic things left that isn't illegal, immoral, fattening, or nasty, and that you can discuss with friends in a public place. So, soak in a soothing bath—even if you're really a shower person at heart! Silken your body with a perfumed oil that matches your mood. Gesture gracefully with perfectly groomed hands and feet.

COME CLEAN

First, there's the bath. Years ago—in fact, longer ago than I would like to remember—I received my first bottle of bubble bath. It was a container of Little Lady, a kiddies' toiletry that predated Tartine and Chocolat and Guerlain's new children's fragrance by several decades. The label had a picture of a small child in a blue dress, and the brown liquid, when poured into the tub, made a wonderful froth of bubbles that transformed my bath into something very special. I became a bath person on the spot.

Since then I have had many special baths. I was initiated into the mysteries of steam baths and *savon beldi* by Khadijah in a blue-and-white-tiled Moroccan *hammam*. I've bathed in an amber-colored tannic-acid lake with five waterfalls cascading into it near Angel Falls in Venezuela. I've relished spa soaks in Bermuda, Mexico, the Caribbean, and beyond. I've been washed in the sacred waters of the Yoruba of Brazil and cleansed in the waters of Mother Africa and soaked in enough bubbles and oils to float the Queen Elizabeth II. Winter or summer, spring or fall, my friends know that if they call me after eleven o'clock in the evening, they're likely to hear the splash of water, for I'll be in the bath. It's the first step to the body beautiful. Before we draw a fragrant tub, though, repeat after me the creed of Bathers Anonymous: If you want to get clean, take a shower. If you want to relax, be calmed and transported to another place, take a bath!

First decide what kind of bath you want to take. There are baths for relaxation, for invigoration, for meditation, and for more. Most of us come to baths for relaxation.

Citrus Soak

This bath, with its hint of bubbles and its citrus aroma, is excellent for winding down before bed.

    2   tablespoons light safflower oil
    ½   cup unscented pure castile shampoo
    4   drops lemon essential oil
    4   drops grapefruit essential oil
    4   drops lime essential oil

Mix the ingredients together in a stoppered bottle and leave them for two or three days to blend. When ready for your bath, shake the bottle slightly and pour one-third of the amount under the tap of running water. When the tub is full, slip in and soak, enjoying the soothing aroma of the citrus fruits and their calming properties.

—— ✿ ——

Cleo's Milk Bath

Cleopatra of Egypt was also an admirer of bathing and is known to have taken milk baths to soothe her skin. Milk baths were popular in the ancient world and can easily be duplicated today.

1 quart whole milk, or the equivalent amount of powdered milk

Add the milk to a tub of warm, bath-temperature water and swirl it around. If this is too rich for your blood, you can also take a milk bath with powdered milk. Simply add enough powdered milk to the running water to make one quart of milk. Milk is soothing and a great treatment for rough or sensitive skin.

The best way to keep healthy skin is to alternate using bubble baths and milk baths with using bath oils and herbal baths, which are just as scented and relaxing. These have the extra benefits of being super body smoothers and simple to make.

—— ✿ ——

Glorious Grenadan Bath Oil

Grenada, in the Caribbean, is known as the spice island. Simply setting foot on the island, you notice the scents of cinnamon, clove, and bay wafting to you on tropical breezes. If you arrive on a cruise ship, you will be greeted by women with small spice baskets containing fresh spices. It's impossible not to buy. Whether you make it to Grenada or not, the scent of the island can be as close as your spice rack.

¼ cup sesame oil	1 large bay leaf, crumbled
2 sticks cinnamon	1 dash nutmeg
6 whole cloves	

Place all the ingredients in a stoppered bottle and allow them to steep for at least one week. When ready to use, strain the spices out with a metal strainer and pour the oil into the tub. This recipe makes enough for one bath, but as the recipe improves with age, you may wish to make a larger amount at one time.

Note: The sesame oil called for here and in all the recipes in this book is ordinary sesame oil that can be obtained at health-food stores, not the nutty-flavored dark sesame oil that is used in Chinese cooking.

Mogul Princess Bath Oil

The scent of sandalwood evokes the courts of Mogul India as no other fragrance can. In the Rajasthan palaces at Jaipur, Udaipur, and Jodhpur, carved sandalwood chests and furniture scent the air with a fragrance that has lasted for centuries.

- 3 tablespoons sesame oil
- 5 drops sandalwood essential oil
- 2 drops amber oil
- 1 drop patchouli oil

Mix the ingredients together in a stoppered bottle and allow them to sit overnight. When ready for the bath, pour the mixture into the tub. Then, sit back and enjoy the luxury of the bath.

Bath salts offer yet another option for the confirmed bather.

Dancer's Soak

Anyone who knows a dancer or anyone who depends on her legs all day knows about Epsom salts. They're the classic bath salt. However, even they take on a more restful aura when they're mixed up with a few drops of relaxing pine oil.

½ cup Epsom salts   5 drops pine oil

Add the Epsom salts to the bath as the tub is filling. When it is almost full, add the pine oil and turn the taps on full to mix it well. Sink in and feel your tense muscles loosen up. The pine oil is stimulating and invigorating. Close your eyes and pretend that you're floating in a pine tree–edged pool in the middle of a primeval forest.

Baño por Yemanja

While bath salts are usually used in secular fashion, the secular and the spiritual come together in this bath for Yemanja, the Yoruba

oriṣa of salt water. In Yorubaland, which crosses the borders of
what today are Nigeria and Benin, Yemanja is the *oriṣa* of the Ogun
River. She is the archetypical mother, nurturing and kind. With the
transatlantic slave trade, many Yoruba people came to the Western
Hemisphere and, miraculously, the religion was maintained. In the
crossing of the Atlantic, Yemoja became Yemaya in Cuba, Iemanja
or Yemanja in Brazil, and Yemanja in the barrios, ghettos, and sub-
urbs of the United States. She grew in stature and in importance
and became the *oriṣa* of salt water, the selfsame salt water that had
granted passage to all those who arrived on these shores from elsewhere. For this, she is saluted in great festivals in places as far-flung
as Cuba, Trinidad, New York, and Salvador da Bahia, Brazil, where
February 2 is her feast day. In Rio de Janeiro, believers and skeptics
alike flock to the beaches on New Year's Eve to honor her with sea-
side altars and offerings in the sand. She is praised with the word
Odoia!

This bath celebrates Yemanja and her power. It is an excellent
one for meditation, as it transforms your bathroom into the waters
of Yemanja, the amniotic fluid of our primal mother.

¼ pound rock salt

1 tub warm water

7 candles in various shades of blue and green

7 bowls (crystal or blue glass or pottery) filled with sand

Add the rock salt to the water. Make sure that it is well dissolved
and well mixed. Place the candles in bowls filled with sand in
strategic places around the tub and light them. Enter the bath rev-
erently; then sit and soak. Relax and listen to the sound of waves
in your mind.

Infusing herbs and other items in the bathwater allows for even more variation in bathing. Bath bags are a useful way to infuse herbs into the bathwater. Actually, bath bags are just a fancy name for large muslin tea bags that allow the herbs and spices to permeate the water with their fragrance and their soothing properties. Lavender is a natural. It has a wonderful fresh scent that is used in aromatherapy as a calming and soothing fragrance. It's also a natural disinfectant. Bergamot brings freshness and clarity, while a sprig or two of rosemary adds a fantastic perfume to the water and can soothe arthritic joints. Needless to say, there is nothing quite like the fragrance of highly scented rose petals. In fact, if you're feeling particularly down, forget the bath bag and simply sprinkle some fragrant rose petals directly into the tub. They'll be a pain to clean out at the end of the bath, but by that time you'll be calm and relaxed.

Oatmeal Bath Baggies

Oatmeal is internationally known for its skin-enhancing properties. It soothes and can also be used as a delicate abrasive to scrub away impurities and slough the skin. It is particularly good for oily skin.

½ yard fine muslin   ¾ pound oatmeal

Sew four or five small rectangular bags about 2¼ inches by 3 inches out of muslin. Leave one end of each bag open, and fill each of the bags with oatmeal. When you get ready to bathe, place a bag under the tap of the running water, allowing the water to run through the bag. The oatmeal will mix with the water as it flows into the tub, softening the water. The bag will keep the oatmeal from clogging your tub, so that you'll get all the benefits of the oatmeal without having your bathtub look like a giant porridge bowl.

Alternately, you can make the bags slightly larger so that you can fit your hand into them. Then, using the filled bag as a mitt, rub it all over your body. You'll be removing the impurities from your skin as you scrub and soak.

Yucca or Spanish bayonet grows wild in parts of the southwestern United States and in Mexico, where it's called *amole.* The roots of the plant have long been used to keep skin smooth and as a soap by Native American peoples. Simply place some pieces of the plant's roots into the bath bags. The root pieces can also be used directly in water as a natural sudser.

Herbal tea bags should not be ignored in the bath. Not only will the hot tea cleanse your system, the same tea bags, or the same herbs in a bath bag, will give your body similar benefits. Peppermint is invigorating. Chamomile is soothing to the nerves and softens the skin. The ancient Egyptians held chamomile in great reverence and used it in body oils to relieve aches and pains.

Botanical Baths

If you live near a store that sells botanical products or have a yard or window garden where you can grow herbs like lavender, lemon verbena, and rose geranium, they too make for a wonderful bath. You can use the herbs in a bath bag or use one of the following methods.

Garden Soak

METHOD I

Pour one cup of boiling water over two tablespoons of the plant product to be used. (You can also use this method with solid botanicals such as strawberries and cucumbers. Puree them first in a blender, then pour the water over them. If using dry herbs, crumble them.) Let the mixture steep for fifteen to twenty minutes; then strain out the liquid and pour it into your tub.

M E T H O D   I I

> Place the plant product to be used in one cup of cider vinegar
> (or one cup of white wine). Let the mixture steep overnight. Then
> strain, and pour the liquid into the tub.

Oil Baths

Women around the world have found that an oil bath from time to time promotes beautiful skin. As I traveled around the world and visited with various women of color, I found that the method changed only slightly: the only real difference in oil baths was the type of oil used. You can try these baths before soaking in a warm tub, or if you're fortunate enough to have a health club with a steam bath, the following baths are great ways to get the best benefits from it.

Mothers in Senegal and Mali rub their newborn babies with shea butter (which is called *karité* in French-speaking Africa) to form their features and to ensure that they have strong limbs. Then they use the shea butter on themselves. Shea butter used to be difficult to find in the United States. Today, with increasing numbers of African immigrants (who use it not only for cosmetic purposes, but also for consumption), it is more readily available. It can be found in bulk in some herb stores.

West African Oil Bath

¼ cup melted *karite* or shea butter (more if necessary)

> *Note: Karité* butter melts very rapidly. Do not attempt to melt it in a
> microwave. Watch it closely as you melt it on the stove.
>
> Wash with hot water, using your usual soap and scrubber to
> make sure that you have cleansed the skin thoroughly. Take half of

the melted shea butter and vigorously rub it over your legs and torso, massaging away aches and pains and molding muscles and joints. Take the remaining butter and massage it into your arms, hands, and neck. Don't worry if it gets into your hair—it promotes hair growth as well. Spend some time working the oil into the vertebrae of your spinal column and your back muscles as though you were rubbing in soap. If you're not limber enough, don't despair; just find a friend to rub it in. Finally, rinse off the excess oil under a warm to hot shower. This will also help the oil to be absorbed. Continue again to massage your entire body and, at the end of the massage, gently massage your face with your fingers, which will still be slightly oily. Take a final rinse with cool to cold water; then pat dry with a towel and go straight to bed. You'll awaken to find that your skin is smooth and you feel as though you have been massaged by a thousand angels.

Africa is not the only continent to have discovered the multiple benefits of a beautifying and relaxing oil bath. Interestingly, in almost all cases, the oil used for bathing is also the primary cooking oil of the region: olive oil in the Mediterranean, gingelly oil in India, and shea butter in West Africa. Women of color throughout the world have traditionally found multiple uses for the ingredients and items that they have on hand.

Indian Oil Bath

In India, many women take oil baths regularly to keep their skin soft and silky. There, the traditional oil of preference is gingelly or sesame oil. This is not the nutty-flavored sesame oil that is sold in Asian grocery stores, but rather the sesame oil that can be found in health-food stores. It's clear and virtually odorless but has great emollient properties.

½ cup sesame oil

Once a week, rub the sesame oil all over your body. Massage the body completely to rub the oil in. Then sit on a towel-covered chair in your bathroom or bedroom and read from your favorite book while the oil is absorbed. Dab off any drips so that you don't ruin the carpet or the furniture. When you've waited for about half an hour, draw yourself a warm bath and get into it with your favorite scrubber. Scrub yourself while you soak and remove the remnants of the oil. When you emerge from the bath, your skin will be silky, soft, and well moisturized.

Hammams and Other Steam Baths

While oil baths restore the skin's natural glow, steam baths allow the skin to breathe and to rid itself of impurities. Think of the multicentury history of North Africa's *hammams,* where patrons leave feeling refreshed physically and cleansed spiritually as well. There is, though, one note of caution. People with heart conditions should not partake without the specific recommendation of their physician. Once you get the okay, though, don't waste a minute before enjoying the refreshing qualities of a good sweat! People tend to confuse steam baths with saunas, but the sensation of dry heat is very different from that of moist heat. Try both, then decide on your personal favorite. Mine is the wet heat of a steam bath or *hammam.*

On the 494th night, Scheherazade said, "And your town will not be truly perfect until it has a *hammam.*" In the *hammam,* the religious and the secular mix and mingle inextricably. You leave feeling cleansed in body and spirit. The word *Saha,* said upon leaving the baths, means "May the bath be beneficial." Anyone who has ever had a *hammam* knows that it is.

The Islamic world is not the only world knowledgeable about the virtues of the bath, and particularly of steam. Many Native American communities use sweat lodges and steam huts to purify body and mind. The *Kama Sutra* defines bathing rituals and recognizes the sensual possibilities of water. Japanese communal soaking tubs are legendary. Bathing is so much a part of the national ethos that some tourist attractions feature cable cars of bathtubs—so that visitors can enjoy the scenery and a soak at the same time!

You cannot truly re-create a steam bath in your home. If you shut the doors and windows and let the hot water run full blast, however, you will have a hint of the steam and why it is so enticing. Sit and enjoy while waiting for the bathwater to cool down enough for you to bathe.

Spiritual Baths

In many cultures, the link between bathing and spirituality is still maintained in baths designed to honor certain deities, to create certain moods, or to celebrate certain events. These baths use natural additives such as herbs and grasses to strengthen and nourish the bather. Many years ago, I was taken to the Mercado Sonora, also called the Mercado de las Curanderas, in Mexico City. I was astonished to recognize many of the herbs and grasses that I knew from botanicas (Hispanic herb shops) in New York City. In addition, there were wonderful new items harking back to that country's Aztec heritage, like the copal incense that was used to perfume the temples. My biggest surprise was finding that the African religion known in the Spanish-speaking world as Santeria was also present. I even got a recipe for an Oşun bath.

Oşun Bath I

Oşun is the Yoruba *orişa* of fresh water, love, beauty, and coquetry. More than her mother and older sister Yemanja, Oşun is associated with the idea of bathing, and her spiritual baths are designed to pull love, money, and sweet things into your life. Taking one of these baths does not depend on your being a committed Yoruba practitioner. Rather, it depends on your willingness to trust the loving powers of Oşun. To bring love into your life, try the following bath.

The ingredients are available at most botanicas. You've got to ask for the ingredients in Spanish or you may not get the same things.

5 fragrant yellow roses	*Esencia attractiva*
Paraíso	*Esencia dominante*
Cloves	*Esencia vente conmigo*
Cinnamon	*Esencia vencedora*
Honey	5 yellow candles
Esencia de amor	

The roses and the *paraíso,* which is a plant, are placed together in a very large saucepan of water, along with the cloves, cinnamon, and honey. Bring the mixture to a boil over medium heat; then lower the heat and continue to simmer for an hour to infuse all the herbs and spices. After the first half hour, add the *esencias* and continue to simmer for the remaining time until they have all mixed well. Divide the mixture among five jars and allow them to cool to room temperature. (If you wish to stay within Oṣun's favorite range of colors, place the mixture in amber-colored jars.) Then each night for five consecutive nights, go into the bathroom and light a yellow candle that you have placed in a yellow or white ceramic or brass bowl. Pour one jar of the mixture into your bath, get in and soak. As the candle burns, invoke Oṣun and her powers and ask her to open you up to love in your life.

Oṣun Bath II

An American version of the Oṣun bath makes use of things that you already have in the house to "sweeten up" you and your environment for love. Five is Oṣun's mystical number, and this bath calls for you to hit your cupboards and your dresser in search of everything sweet in your house.

- 5 drops each of five sweetening agents in the house, from honey to brown sugar to Equal
- 5 drops each of five body lotions, perfumes, bath oils, colognes, essential oils, and so forth
- 5 drops each of five alcoholic beverages that are open
- 1 small bottle of a pilsner-type beer (or if you're going for a big love, 1 small bottle of champagne)
- 5 drops ammonia

Place all the ingredients together in a large basin. (If you have a golden-colored brass basin, you're absolutely on the money.) Fill the basin with cold water. Get into the tub with the basin, and while invoking the powers of Oṣun, pour the contents over your head. As you pour the contents over yourself, ask Oṣun for what you want aloud. Blot yourself dry and go to bed after meditating on your wishes.

When I asked my friend Ayo what to do about the wet hair, she replied curtly, "Wear a turban, a head tie, or a hat for five days!" I asked her if the effort was really worth all of that. She replied with a serious cat-that-got-the-cream look that let me know that this bath had done wonders for her. "The bath," she explained, "is an attracting bath. And when you use it, you have to fight the folk off." Sounded good to me.

SOAPS, SCRUBS, AND SO FORTH

The water in which we bathe is only one element of the bath. There are also the soaps, the scrubs, and the manner in which we dry ourselves. I'm not only a bath oil and bubble bath collector, but also a soap collector. If I spot a new one on a trip, it's sure to find its way into my suitcase and back home to my bathroom in Brooklyn, where I jokingly say that I have the world's largest collection of bubbles and soap and the world's smallest claw-foot bathtub. I've always loved different soaps.

Soaps have been around for millennia. The first soaps came from a mixture of the fats of sacrificial animals and the ashes of the fires in which they had been sacrificed. There were other methods for cleansing as well. In North and South America, plants like soapwort and soap weed were used. The Egyptians employed a mixture of fine sand and fragrant oils to cleanse themselves—an excellent exfoliant even today. Arabs used perfumed clay, which inspired these lines:

> *'Twas in the bath, a piece of perfumed clay*
> *Came from my loved one's hand to mine, one day.*
> *"Art thou, then, musk or ambergris," I said,*
> *"that by thy scent my soul is ravished?"*
> *"Not so," it answered, "Worthless earth was I,*
> *But long I kept the rose's company:*
> *Thus near its perfect fragrance to me came,*
> *Else I'm but earth, the worthless and the same."*

A similar type of perfumed clay is still in use as a soap in areas of North Africa today. It's the *tafal* of Tunisia. There, it is a black clay soap, which is placed in the sun in large bronze pots and covered with rose petals or wild geranium flowers. Later, it's diluted down with orange-flower water. The clay soap actually comes from Morocco, where it is sold already diluted and perfumed in large vats in the markets. The French who live there call it *savon beldi*. It has the consistency and look of brown Jell-O, but it makes your skin feel as though you've just put it on for the first time. Whenever I go to Morocco, I travel with a large Tupperware container so that I can bring back some of this wonderful soap.

There are all manner of soaps: African soaps where ash, papaya, and fat are blended together in a grainy mixture that is sold in round balls in the markets of West Africa; Brazilian soaps that smell of caramelized sugar and are made from fresh bee's honey. Bee's honey is also an ingredient in a honey-and-jasmine soap from China. Honey, all by itself, is a major ingredient in some Yoruba Oṣun baths. The Yoruba also prepare a soap that is the color of blackstrap molasses. It is strong and stings the skin slightly when used, but it is also soft and leaves the skin more lustrous. This black soap is more than soap to many New World Yoruba. For them, it has ritual meaning and is an important link to the Old World of Africa. The soap, imported from Africa, is so full of meaning and significance that it is used in Yoruba initiation rituals in areas of the Americas where the Yoruba religion has been maintained.

I can remember as a child being in my grandmother Harris's kitchen in the projects in Jamaica, New York, when she made soap. Grandma Harris, a transplanted southerner, was not happy unless she had a small plot of land to grow things on, good gospel music, and, of course, her own freshly made soap. I'll never forget the smells, the large pot steaming on the back of the stove, and the cries of, "Get back, child, you'll burn yourself. Don't you know that's lye!" I will also never forget the feeling of bathing with the simple brown cake of pure homemade soap. It was not at all like the Ivory and perfumed soaps that my mother had in the bathroom, or the bar of Octagon soap with which Grandma Harris did her laundry. That was the beginning of my love for soap. I've never gone as far as my grandmother—time, trouble, and fear of working with lye have kept me from attempting to make my own soap. I do feel, however, that that small brown slab marked me for life.

I still think of soap as one of life's affordable luxuries. When I want a new perfume but really shouldn't spend on it, I'll enjoy its fragrance by buying a bar of the soap. Soap is also one of the few things that lasts virtually forever, although the scent may diminish. Interestingly, it's also one of the few things that is better after being stored. The soap hardens slightly over time and will then last longer once you begin using it. You can enjoy the soap and get the benefit of its scent even before you lather up by storing it in your lingerie drawer. I always keep a few bars of soap in mine, and the rest go into a large Ghanaian basket in my bathroom to perfume the air.

Soap, though, is not the only equipment that you'll need for a perfect bath. The well-dressed bathroom today has as many accessories and gadgets as the kitchen. I find, however, that you don't need expensive whirlpool attachments and shower nozzles, or radios to sing along with, to enjoy the luxury of a perfect bath. A few simple items will make your bath more enjoyable and you more beautiful.

Take a hint from my friend Theodora. When I stayed at her house in Abidjan, I noticed that the bathroom always had a small piece of blue-string fishnet hanging over the shower faucets. When I asked, she said that it was a *filet,* a net. She added, "They're not from here, but at home in Benin we use them to wash with." Several years later, when I went to Benin, my curiosity got the best of me and I headed off to the Dan Tokpa market, where I found aisle upon aisle of vendors selling the same *filets* I'd seen at Theodora's. (They were almost all blue, but you could find a few white ones if you tried.) You simply purchase a piece and cut it into the length you desire. Needless to say, I bought some and stuffed them into my suitcase, which was already bulging with Yoruba black soap, African fabric in myriad designs and colors, and a few masks for good measure. It took me a month or so to find the *filets* when I got back to the States. But then, I cut off a piece and took it with me into the bath and used it instead of a washcloth. It was wonderful: just abrasive enough to stimulate the skin but not rough enough to scratch. Over the years, I've been husbanding my small piece of *filet*. (It's easier to pack on business trips than a loofah or brush.) Next time I'm buying a larger piece.

Theodora's Filet

If you live in an area where you can find cotton fishing net, you can make your own *filet*. Just cut a small piece. Wet it and give it a test to make sure that it is not too abrasive. Use it and enjoy.

Gant de Toilette

Whenever I'm in Martinique, Guadeloupe, or France, I always make a beeline for a department store to stock up on *gants de toilette,* which are my favorite facecloths. They're exactly like American washcloths, with one vital difference: they're in the form of mitts. I like being able to fit my hand inside it. When my supply runs out and I'm not heading to the French Caribbean or France, I make them easily. You can too.

1 washcloth   Matching thread

Find a washcloth that is large enough for your hand to fit into the rectangle made when it is folded double. Then double the washcloth and sew a small seam up the long side and one of the short sides. You'll be left with a mitt that will fit over your hand. Turn it inside out. *Voilà, votre gant de toilette!*

Remember, with your *gant de toilette* or any facecloth, they must be kept scrupulously clean. It's not weird to think of changing your facecloth daily. Do as I do and buy plain white cloths for the face and colors for the body; then you'll always know which is your facecloth. To get them really clean, do what my hairdresser, Sandy, does with all her clothes: add a few pieces of lemon to each washing-machine load, or adopt the old-fashioned method of boiling them once a month in water to which you've added a few drops of lemon juice or vinegar. If you've been truly negligent (and I am occasionally), try this old-fashioned mixture to freshen them up again: soak the facecloths overnight in a mixture of water and white vinegar; then wash as usual. The cloths will be ready for use again.

Occasionally, our skin just seems a bit dull and drab. That's when you need a body scrub to rev up your circulation. These light abrasives help slough off the dead skin and therefore make the skin glow.

Women of color from traditional cultures use many different scrubs and exfoliants to enhance their beauty. In southern India and among the Indian communities in Trinidad, Martinique, and Guadeloupe, brides are "marinated" in turmeric paste before the wedding. The paste, which is made of turmeric and water, is ceremonially slathered on the bride to purify her. The mixture is left on the skin for an hour or longer, and is thought to soften and smooth the skin. Turmeric paste is also believed to restrict hair growth. Sound good? There's one downside to consider before you head off to your kitchen in search of turmeric. The paste stains the bride and everything else that it touches with a slightly saffron tint. While this is considered attractive and indeed auspicious in parts of the Indian world, it may not be the best thing for you.

---- ✻ ----

Yvette's Egyptian Salt Rub

Aristocratic ancient Egyptians used a mixture of fine white sand and perfumed oils as an exfoliant cleanser. My formerly peripatetic cousin, Yvette, assures me that modern ones use salt in much the same way.

¼ cup coarse table salt

Wet yourself all over. Then, standing in the tub, pour a handful of salt into your palm. Rub the salt on the dull areas of your body, using slow circular movements. Avoid any nicks or cuts you may have on your body or you will truly understand the expression "to rub salt into the wound." When finished, complete the rub with an invigorating cool shower.

---- ✻ ----

Sugar Scrape

Among the traditional peoples who live around the Mediterranean basin, the olive is the staff of life. It is the oil in oil lamps, the cooking oil of choice, the hair conditioner, and the emollient of the region. This sugar scrape gives those of us outside the region an approximation of the olive oil and abrasive glove treatment of many *hammams.*

¼ cup olive oil
¼ cup sugar

Pouring a bit at a time into the palm of your hand, coat your entire body with a thin film of olive oil. Then take a small handful of sugar and scrape it across the skin, using slow circular movements. Continue in this manner until you have used up the sugar. Concentrate on elbows, knees, and other notorious trouble spots. When finished, shower off the residue with a tepid shower.

Down-Home Mayo Scrub

Among African Americans, the kitchen has supplied many traditional beauty items. This recipe for sloughing off dead skin uses mayonnaise and cornmeal. The mayonnaise is especially moisturizing, so this is a good slougher for dry skin.

¼ cup mayonnaise   ¼ cup cornmeal

Slather a thin film of mayonnaise all over the body. Then take a small palmful of cornmeal and scrape it over the body, using slow circular movements. Continue until you have used all the cornmeal. When finished, rinse off thoroughly under a shower, making sure that you have removed all the cornmeal. If you don't, you'll feel as though you just left a sandy beach.

Alternately, if you have oily skin and do not wish to use the mayonnaise, simply wet the skin and then use the cornmeal. Once again, be sure to rinse well. Should any of these scrubs become a regular part of your beauty ritual (don't abuse them; certainly no more than once a week), then you may wish to keep a container in your bathroom filled with your abrasive of choice: salt, sugar, or cornmeal.

Sloughers and exfoliants will bring a glow to the entire body, but what about the peskier elbows, knees, and heels? My mother has always had a solution for that one.

Elbows-on-the-Table Lemon Rub

While it's not polite to sit with your elbows on the table, that's the only way that you can get the true benefits of this treatment.

1 large lemon, cut in half

Place each elbow into a lemon half and simply sit with your elbows on the table. It may not be polite, but it is smoothing, and over time it bleaches dark, scaly elbows.

An alternative to my mother's treatment is one that I learned from my West African friend Fatou.

Fatou's Elbow Brightener

1 lemon
2 tablespoons table salt

Cut the lemon in half and sprinkle a tablespoon of salt on one half. Over a sink or in the tub, rub the lemon half over your elbow in slow movements, as though you were trying to juice it, for five minutes or longer. Repeat on the other elbow, using the other lemon half.

While lemons may be miraculous for bleaching for some of us, in Mexico they turn to the ubiquitous avocado for almost everything. A trip to the market explains why. Whether in Acapulco or Mexico City, in Ixtapan de la Sal or Ixtapa, avocados are staples in Mexican markets. Piled up in Toltec pyramids of deep green globes with a square incision cut out of one to reveal the creamy pale green and yellow interior, they are the country's miracle fruit. They turn up in traditional recipes for facial masques, hair tonics, and, naturally, body scrubs.

Avocado Scrub

As you saw in the preceding chapter, this works on the face as well as the body.

1 avocado

Peel the avocado and eat it. What you want for this recipe is the peel. How's that for ecologically sound! Rub the peel of the avocado over rough areas like elbows and knees. The inside of the peel contains soothing avocado oil that will gradually soften the skin. Because the peel is slightly abrasive, it will smooth the skin as well.

FINISHING OFF

Drying off after bathing is an essential part of the process. Towels are a relatively recent invention in the Western world. They're still unknown in many parts of the traditional world of tropical women of color. There, the sun dries you off naturally. After bathing, one simply dresses in one's fresh clothing. Sticky, you might think. Indeed, so did I until I tried it in Bahia, Brazil. It was surprisingly refreshing. The all-cotton clothing blotted up the moisture, and what residual moisture was left after the first few minutes was cooling rather than cloying. It's not something that really works for us in northern climes, but when dressing in light clothing in a very warm climate, it's wonderful. Those of us who live in cooler areas should stick to our Western towels. Just look for the thickest, most absorbent towels that you can find. If you really become a bath aficionado, splurge on a terry robe. There's nothing to match the sensation of stepping out of the bath into a welcoming terry robe and lightly patting yourself dry all over.

Once dry, it's time to moisturize. Oiling the body with sweet-smelling unguents after bathing is a tradition that goes back to the Egyptians. While upper-class Egyptians were using perfumed sand to scrub with, the proletariat was rubbing down with palm oil. The orange-hued oil is still the body oil of choice in many parts of West Africa. It stains everything an orangy tint that is considered quite beautiful. The use of palm oil as a body oil has also crossed the Atlantic; in northeastern Brazil, many attribute the beautiful complexions of the women of color to its use. It's a great emollient.

In other parts of West Africa, shea butter or *karité* is used for oiling the body. A natural vegetable product, shea butter has a strong odor. I know because when my friend Theodora found some for me in the market at Treicheville, Abidjan, I wrinkled my nose in despair. She showed me how it is prepared for cosmetic use. The round white balls of the vegetable butter are placed in a saucepan with aromatic herbs or spices. You can use everything from lavender to cloves, depending on your personal preferences. The oil is heated until it becomes liquid and then cooked with the herbs for about half an hour until the scent of the herbs has been absorbed. The liquid is allowed to cool slightly and then poured into a container before it hardens again. When it returns to its solid form, it has been deodorized and rescented with the refreshing aroma of the herbs. In this manner it is used for everything from rubbing down scaly legs to massaging the stomachs of pregnant women. Daily massages with *karité* are believed to prevent stretch marks!

In the South Seas, fragrant coconut oil scented with frangipani is known as *tiare* and used as a body oil, while in parts of southern India, gingelly or sesame oil reigns supreme.

HANDS AND FEET

You'd be surprised what your hands say about you. How many times have you looked at a person and thought that he or she had artistic hands, pianist's hands, working hands, or simply unkempt hands.

Hands and feet, too, are more expressive than most of us think. Their care, or neglect, tells a lot about you. Once, after a television appearance at an ungodly hour of the morning, I was delighted to receive a letter from a friend, who wrote to tell me that as she was emerging from her cocoon of sleep, she had switched on the television set and seen a familiar pair of hands—mine! She recognized them by the way I used them.

In ancient China, it was easy to identify a person of gentility because the fingernails were allowed to grow to extreme lengths. The fragile nails were covered with golden nail guards, which were frequently encrusted with precious jewels.

Brides in traditional families in Egypt, North Africa, the Middle East, and India have their hands and feet painted with henna in intricate weblike designs in a ceremony called the *mehandi*. In Egypt, wedding guests are given henna to hold in the palms of their hands during the ceremony. It is thought that the henna-stained palms bring good luck. In Tunisia, a small heart or other design is painted on the palm of the hand at ceremonial gatherings. The use of henna on hands and feet is not only ceremonial; it is also thought to prevent perspiration.

Henna, which is mainly known to us in the West as a hair cosmetic, is said to be good for skin by women in North Africa and Islamic countries. There is a tradition in the Islamic world that says that the prophet Mohammed wanted to see all women with hennaed hands. It is recounted that he once saw a woman with unhennaed hands and commented that she should not neglect her hands to the extent that they looked like a man's. Needless to say, that woman hennaed her hands until the day she died. Another tale of the Prophet and henna has it that he taught his daughter, Fatima, to apply special henna designs to her hands and feet so that he would be able to know when she was menstruating without her having to tell him. Whatever the origins of henna's use as an adornment for hands, the designs are spectacular. In India, North Africa, and much of the Middle East, the designs are delicate arabesques of swirling black. Some even feature verses in Arabic script. One such verse expresses the wearer's pride: "It is not the dye that has adorned my hands; it is my hands that have enhanced the dye."

I remember badgering Thiane to take me to get my hands and feet done one day in Senegal. "We'll have to stop at the market first," she said. We went to the stall with burlap bags full of a light greenish powder that I was told was the henna. Thiane then asked in Wolof for an additional powder. "This will help the henna blacken more rapidly," she explained. We gathered our packages and headed off.

In Dakar's medina, at the home of the friend who was going to apply the henna, we began the process. First, Thiane and her friend cut stencils out of adhesive tape and arranged them on my hands and feet. "We're just doing simple designs so that it doesn't take as much time," they explained. They then combined the henna and the black powder with water into a mudlike mixture and applied it to my hands and feet. "This is not the traditional way," they informed me, as they encased my hands and feet in plastic bags, "but it helps the henna to darken quickly. Otherwise, you'd have to stay here for twenty-four hours." I sat with hands and feet stretched out in front of me in their plastic bags trying to think of like tortures. The minutes snailed by like days. The hours turtled by like centuries. Finally, after about three hours, they liberated me.

I held my breath as they undid the plastic bags and declared me "done." We gradually peeled off the adhesive tape and revealed a pattern of diamonds in my palms and at the edge of each finger. The color was a deep black, with reddish hennalike edges. My feet boasted black soles and a booteelike scalloped edging. I was thrilled, and ever since, time notwithstanding, I get my hands and feet hennaed at each possible opportunity.

⚜

Senegalese Stenciled Hands

Senegalese women use a stencil method that is a bit simpler than the Moroccan one.

2 ounces black henna

¼ pint hot water

1 roll wide adhesive tape

2 plastic baggies, large enough to fit over the hands

This is not a do-it-yourself project. You'll need a willing friend, either to try her hand as designer or to allow you to experiment on her. Cleanse the hands thoroughly. You may want to do a manicure next. Since henna is a dye, any snipping, pushing, and cutting that are done afterwards will have an effect on the design once it is in place.

Mix the henna and the hot water in an earthenware, glass, or enamel bowl with a wooden spoon. (Do not use a metal bowl or spoon, as it will react with the henna.) Take a few minutes to test the henna to make sure that your friend has no adverse reaction to it. Then, decide on the design that you will do and cut a stencil of it from the wide adhesive tape. Try a simple design like circles or stars. (Theodora, my Beninese friend, raves about the time she saw a Senegalese courtesan with clubs, hearts, spades, and diamonds hennaed onto the palms of her hands.) Remember that the henna will dye any part of the hands not covered by the adhesive. Set the stencils in place, and then tape up the areas of the hands that you do not wish to dye. Now, apply the henna paste. When finished, encase the hands in the plastic baggies, tie them loosely, and instruct your friend to remain immobile as long as possible. The

longer she can wait, the darker and longer-lasting the designs will
be. If possible, leave the baggies on several hours. When ready, remove the baggies, peel off the henna, and voilà—Senegalese stenciled hands.

Remember, with the stencil method, you can henna only the
area you wish to. If you don't want to dye your entire palm, you can
give yourself a henna ring or a small henna star. Experiment.

Marvelous Moroccan Hennaed Hands

It's a tedious task and one that you cannot do yourself, as working
on your own hand is an impossible task. If you have the patience,
artistic ability, and a willing friend, however, the results can be
stunning. Begin slowly with a small design.

2 ounces red or black henna

¼ pint hot water

1 pointed orange stick to use as an applicator

Proceed as with the Senegalese Stenciled Hands. When the henna
is ready, take the orange stick, dip it into the henna, and have your
friend draw the outline of a simple design on your right hand. Be
careful, because if you stray from the line or smudge, you've got to
quickly wipe it off and begin again. (If you're truly timid, begin with
the soles of your feet. That way, if you make mistakes, only you and
she will know.) The person who is having the designs done has to
sit with her hands or feet immobile for the time that it takes the
henna to dry, so that it doesn't smudge. The one who is doing the
drawing must have a steady hand. Once the design is finished and
dry, wrap the hands or feet in an old piece of terry-cloth toweling.

(Remember, it too will end up henna-stained.) Use your hands or feet as little as possible for the rest of the evening. The following morning, peel off the henna paste to reveal the design in red or black set off against the palms of the hands or soles of the feet.

If henna appeals to you, but you're not sure that you want to dye your hands, try using henna paste as a permanent nail polish.

Henna Nail Polish

This method will give your nails the traditional reddish orange look of henna, which is beautiful when buffed to a high gloss. It's permanent, but if you get tired of it, you can hide it under a few coats of nail polish.

1 ounce red henna	1 small paintbrush
⅛ pint hot water	

Mix the henna and the water in a nonreactive bowl with a wooden spoon. When you have a thin paste, apply it to the nails with the small paintbrush. Allow the paste to dry thoroughly in the sun, remembering that the longer you leave it on the darker it will become. When you're ready, remove the paste and you'll have henna-dyed nails—permanent nail polish that won't chip or peel. You'll also be able to monitor your nail growth, as the new nail will grow out undyed.

Remember that nails, like hair, grow slowly. Don't just sit there bemoaning your stubby-nailed fate; do something. Nails are an indicator of your complete health. Nails that truly do not grow may indicate other problems and should be checked by a physician. If it's simply that you bite them, or that they're thin and brittle, there are things that can be done. If you're a nail biter, take a tip from breast-feeding African mothers who are ready to wean their children. They rub bitter aloe on their nipples to stop their infants from nursing. Rub a bit of aloe under your nails—you'll stop putting them in your mouth. Once the biting has stopped, help your nails along with a hot oil treatment.

Hot Oil Treatment for Nails

1 small dish of warm olive oil

After cleaning your nails thoroughly and rubbing them with a nail-brush, dip the nails in the warmed olive oil. The oil should be warm enough to feel warm, not hot enough to burn. Remove your hand from the oil and massage each nail individually, rubbing in the olive oil. When you have finished massaging each nail, continue to rub the olive oil into your fingers and hand, knuckle by knuckle, joint by joint. The olive oil promotes nail strength, and the massage will promote nail growth.

Beatriz's Nail Treatment

A variation on this theme comes to me from a Mexican friend. It's stimulating and simple.

¼ cup sweet almond oil
¼ cup freshly squeezed lemon juice

Warm the sweet almond oil slightly, place it in a saucer, and dip in your fingernails. Massage the oil into the hands and the nails, and leave it on for at least five minutes. During that time, gently push the cuticles back with an orange stick and shape the nails with an emery board. When done, blot off the residue with a paper towel. Then rub the nails with the lemon juice to stimulate them and to give them a fresh clean smell.

Anyone who works in a kitchen knows how many unpleasant kitchen odors can cling to the hands. As a devotee of the stinking rose known as garlic and a champion onion eater, I am always on the lookout for ways to rid my hands of strong cooking odors.

Mama's Deodorizing Hand Cleaner

My mother, a whiz at household tricks, came up with this method of getting rid of onion odor.

- ¼ cup cucumber juice
- ½ lemon, freshly squeezed
- 2 tablespoons salt

Mix all the ingredients together and rub the grainy mixture over your hands. Concentrate on the smelly areas. The lemon and cucumber juice will remove the offending odor, and the salt provides a slight abrasive that allows the mixture to get into hard-to-reach areas to really get rid of the scent.

Potato Magic

In India, where garlic is an ingredient in many dishes and where expressive hands are a hallmark of beauty, they have a simple hand-freshening trick that calls for the deodorizing properties of a white potato.

1 small white potato

Cut the potato in half and rub the white side over the hands again and again. The potato removes the odor and is also at work softening the hands.

Far Eastern Hand Freshener

The chrysanthemum is a symbol of autumn in Chinese culture. It is not inconceivable that a woman arranging an autumnal bouquet first noticed that chrysanthemum leaves will remove odors from hands.

4 to 6 chrysanthemum leaves

Crush the fresh chrysanthemum leaves between your fingers and rub them over your hands. The odors will disappear.

Rose geranium leaves also work wonders and leave the hands lightly scented with their splendid fragrance.

_____ ⚜ _____

Carioca Hand Cream

If your hands are rough and need a bit more soothing, take a tip from my Carioca friend Vera. She softens and soothes her hands with a mixture of banana and butter that is good enough to eat. It is especially effective when it is allowed to remain on the hands overnight.

½ banana, very ripe
1½ teaspoons unsalted butter

Peel the banana. Then, in a small saucer, mix the banana and the butter together with the back of a fork until you have a cream. Slather the cream on your hands, working it into each knuckle and joint. Cover them with a pair of old cotton gloves, and go to bed and dream of the beaches of Ipanema.

_____

Hands are funny. As with any part of the body, once you've paid particular attention to them, they just seem to become more graceful. You gesture with them more often and use them to their best advantage. Some of this comes naturally. An exercise that I learned in grammar school from my Indian friend Shika will help you have more graceful fingers.

_____ ⚜ _____

Shika's Finger Exercises

Decades after learning this exercise, on a trip to Madras, India, where we were entertained by *bharata natya* dancers, I would discover that the finger exercises were actually one of the mudras or movements from that ancient art of the dance.

After you've conditioned your fingers, flex them. Then point the thumbs of both hands toward the palms. Follow by closing the fingers, one at a time, over the thumb. Slowly, index . . . third . . . fourth . . . and fifth fingers. Now, beginning with the fifth finger, slowly open them out again like the petals opening on a flower. Rotate your wrists as your fingers move in and out. Continue doing this a few times and I can virtually guarantee that your gestures will become more graceful.

Where the hands go, the feet have got to follow. Don't neglect them. Smooth, baby-soft feet are always beautiful. Dorotea, a friend I met in the Dominican Republic, gave me a hint I never fail to follow every summer. "When near a beach," she said, "don't miss the opportunity to take a long stroll in the sand. Not only is it excellent exercise for the calves and the legs, but the sand's abrasion smoothes away callouses and roughness."

If you're not near a beach, give your feet a good going over with a coarse pumice stone every time you're ready to come out of the bath. The dead skin will be softened by this treatment and will rub away more easily. Then slather them with oil to keep them soft and smooth. All the hand-care recipes that I've given work equally well with the feet. Just remember that if you're slathering on a thick cream or oil before heading to bed, a pair of white cotton socks will help the treatment and will also protect your bed linen. If, like me, you can't always remember to polish all those little piggies, think about using a little henna polish for a permanent glow.

Henna Cooler

Try this idea from India to keep you feeling wonderful. If you're troubled in the summer by hot, sweaty feet, just powder them with henna. Use a colorless henna unless you want to stain the feet. The henna, somehow, cools and freshens the feet.

1 ounce colorless natural henna

Just dust the henna lightly on the feet. This amount should work for several dustings.

Cornstarch Duster

Like the women in India who used the henna that they had on hand to cool their feet, women in the southern United States also use something that is around the house—cornstarch. It's as simple as dusting your feet with it; the cornstarch will absorb the moisture. It's a trick that mothers also use for babies' bottoms to prevent diaper rash.

1 tablespoon cornstarch (more if necessary)

Simply use the cornstarch as you would powder to dust on the feet.

Hot feet are a summer plague; cold feet can be the bane of a winter existence. In the southern United States, the heating power of chile is sometimes put to an unusual use. A sprinkle of cayenne pepper in the bottoms of your stockings is thought to warm up cold tootsies. Don't laugh; it works!

Sometimes, you just want to relax and soak your feet. Many summers ago I learned this soothing herbal soak, which can be prepared with pine needles that you find on a slow walk in the woods.

---- ✤ ----

Pine Pamperer

½ cup pine needles   ½ cup boiling water

Place the pine needles in a small bowl, add the boiling water, and steep for fifteen to twenty minutes. When the needles have yielded up their piney essence, transfer the liquid into a basin large enough to hold both feet. Fill the basin with warm water and soak your feet while thinking of forest glades.

If you don't have time to soak your feet, get a lift by doing just that, lifting your feet. Try resting on a slantboard, or on a bed with several pillows tucked under your feet. Everyone is entitled to a little pampering after a long day. One woman I know usually takes a quick nap in the afternoon. After an hour's nap with her feet elevated, she's ready for anything the evening offers. When you think that your feet spend your lifetime carrying you around, and getting you from place to place despite the abuse heaped upon them, don't they deserve a rest?

POSTURE: THE FINAL TOUCH

Most women of color have fantastic posture. It's the final touch to a beautiful woman. They seem to announce their presence just by entering a room. This, of course, is a very personal attribute, but you can develop some of it by simply throwing back your shoulders and thinking regal thoughts. My five-foot-one, eighty-two-year-old mother could give many of us a lesson in strutting. When she has what I call an Oṣun attack and is dressed up and made up to her satisfaction, she throws her shoulders back and steps out as though she were Naomi Campbell on a runway.

Women in Africa, the Caribbean, and Asia spend much of their lives carrying heavy bundles on their heads. My friend Theodora, when I lived in a fourth-floor walk-up, amazed me one day. She was returning home to West Africa with a suitcase so laden with goodies that we couldn't get it down the narrow stairs. "Help me get it on my head," she said. Horrified, I helped her lift it up onto her head. She rose slowly, straightened her shoulders, and headed down the steps without a second thought, like the empress Anna Nzinga greeting European royalty. I stood on the top step, mouth agape.

Posture Perfecter

While Theodora's load is certainly not recommended, the old tried-and-tested trick of a few books on the head has never harmed a flea. Find a book, place it on your head, and walk. Neck straight, shoulders down, glide . . . that's it. Add a few more books, one at a time. Then go on, girl—strut your stuff. Enter a room like Jessye Norman enters the stage, and descend those stairs like Josephine Baker at the Folies Bergère. Watch the heads turn as you enter a room.

You've worked hard to get your beautiful body; now flaunt it!

☙

Chapter 6

THE BODY ADORNED

Put on that red dress, baby,
'cause we're going out tonight.
TRADITIONAL BLUES

She has an embroidered skirt.
She has cloth from the coast.
She has grace like no one else.
What does a Bahiana have?
DORIVAL CAYMMI

THE SCENT OF VETIVER and the swish of a sari in a light Bombay breeze. The musky aroma of *gongo* wafting from beneath a billowing boubou on a Dakar avenue. The fragrance of roses and the flashing of kohled eyes under a *buibui* in a sun-dappled alleyway in Mombasa. The timeless essence of jasmine and the eternal elegance of a cheongsam (or *chi pao*) turning a corner in Taipei. The perfume of copal and the mystical layers of meaning embroidered into the bodice of a Oaxacan dress in Mexico. Whether in India, Senegal, Kenya, Taiwan, Mexico, or elsewhere in the world, women of color have traditionally dressed in ways that are particularly seductive. Their seductiveness is enhanced by their mastery of ornament and perfume and all of the goddesses' arts that appeal to the senses. Waist beads add a rhythmic clicking to the steps of many a West African woman. Multiple colors and textures set off a Mexicana's beauty. Subtle perfumes and sensuous fabrics highlight the loveliness of our Asian sisters.

The bright light of the tropics in which many of us live leaches the color from pastels, so bright colors and startling combinations are the norm. Brilliant turquoise, shocking pink, citron yellow, acid green, and color couplings that would be unthinkable in northern climes blossom in tropical areas and reveal new visual treats.

We wear our gold, if we've got it. Gold and silver jewelry is traditionally our portable wealth and our safe-deposit box in times of trouble. Any woman treasures a piece of jewelry, whether it is a heavy breastplate of silver encrusted with cabochon stones and enameled designs, a pair of finely filigreed earrings, or a ring of gold-colored straw encircled with colored string. Semiprecious stones add colorful highlights to traditional garments, not the diamonds and rubies of the Western world. Instead, heavy balls of amber are worn in necklaces by the Berber women of Morocco and the Peul/Fulani of Mali. Turquoise pieces highlighted with coral hang around the necks of the Navajo. Jade brings luck and longevity to the Chinese.

The final vestmental touch in many areas is a hat or head scarf that may identify the wearer's age group, family line, clan, or marital status. In some cultures, no self-respecting woman would venture out of her house without the addition of a bit of fragrance, whether it is the stem of jasmine worn tucked into her bun or a dab of vanilla extract behind each ear.

For centuries, women of color around the world have greatly influenced the way we dress. Yet, somehow, ethnic dressing conjures up images of a young woman of dubious cleanliness dressed in faded garments that seem cut from Jacob's coat of many colors. She's bedecked in pieces with clashing cultural symbols and wearing so much jewelry that she seems like a demented nun clicking her beads, and her odor has nothing to do with roses or frangipani. Yes, for many of us the sixties took the thrill out of celebrating the ethnic variety of the world through its clothing.

Let's go back, though, to the true meaning of it all. Think of the luxurious slide of shimmering silk over perfumed skin that is the Chinese *chi pao* or the Vietnamese *ao dai*. Not only does it perfectly highlight the traditional body types of its wearers, it is also comfortable because it is fully lined and undergarments can be minimal. Practical side slits allow for movement while increasing the garment's sensual appeal.

Consider the multiple folds of a silk or cotton sari, which can be worn in a variety of ways, depending on the area of India from which one harks. Moreover, each garment can be worn by all the women of a family regardless of their variations in size and height, because the sari is refashioned to the individual demands of the wearer each time it is worn. Many Indian women own and can still wear saris belonging to their grandmothers.

The boubou, or traditional dress of the women of Senegal, is basically a rectangle of fabric with a neck hole cut in it. Yet the variations that are available through embroidery, neckline changes, and fabric are endless. (Many of the fabrics are designer mill ends from French couture houses.) These multiple color combinations and embroidered designs make the boubou a dress of such elegant simplicity that it has been adopted as formal wear by many West African women.

Mention Salvador da Bahia to people in Brazil and they go into raptures. The Bahiana, or traditional woman of Bahia, is noted for her charm and grace, her cooking, and her traditional dress. A floor-length skirt of brightly printed cotton fabric or pristine embroidered white is worn over several starched petticoats. Accompanying the skirt is a white off-the-shoulder blouse embroidered with openwork lace that highlights her bronzed skin perfectly. Multiple strands of tiny glass beads complete the outfit, which is topped off with an intricately tied turban that identifies her religious affiliations.

Perhaps the one traditional garment with which we are most familiar is the North African caftan. Discovered in the sixties by suburbia, it was found to be perfect for lounging—eternally elegant and supremely comfortable. Made in fabrics ranging from rough wools to delicate cottons to luxurious silks, caftans can go almost everywhere and be in style.

One of the attractions of ethnic dressing is that long before the Western world returned to natural fibers, natural was the exotic woman's password. Fine cottons (and who has yet topped delicate Egyptian cottons?), intricately woven silks enhanced with embroidered patterns, delicate linens, and handwoven wools are the hallmarks of the clothing of the exotic world. The Egyptians and Chinese, though, both thought that wool was "barbarian," and evidenced great distaste for the fabric. In India, the silky hair of the long-haired goat native to the province of Kashmir was and is woven into shawls so fine that they can fit through a wedding ring. They call it *pashmina*, and it is the finest of cashmeres. Linen fabric dates as far back as the Neolithic era, and is mentioned in the Bible. Cooler climates necessitated the use of fur and even the dreaded wool, but they were worn with style and panache. Think of the buckskin dresses of the Sioux decorated with elk teeth and cowrie shells. Designs belonged to particular families and were passed down as legacies from mother to daughter. Think also of Navajo blankets and of the original Inuit anoraks.

Colors hold strong meaning among many peoples. For some of the Plains Indians, yellow represents maturity and perfection; red symbolizes life and is sacred; green stands for evolution and development. In Rajasthan, India, different seasons of the year dictate the wearing of different colors. Blues are worn in the cooler months, while vivid pinks signal the coming of the spring season.

The designers of the Western world have long been seduced by the style of women of color. Ralph Lauren's 1981 Navajo-inspired fall collection created a demand for Native American jewelry of the Southwest that has not yet subsided. Concha belts sprouted on the most unlikely waists; turquoise necklaces complete with *jaclas* hung down from faux maidens' necks; and the whole idea of ethnic dressing was somehow subverted. Ethnic dressing should be a knowing celebration of another culture. Clothing should not simply be purchased for a "look" or a trend, but rather lovingly acquired with knowledge and respect. The style of women of color is eternal and timeless, and it is for all. You don't have to belong to a specific ethnic group to delight in the trappings of its heritage. You should, however, respect the group's culture. Wear nothing ethnic in the area from which it comes unless you wish to pay tribute to your hosts and they have granted you permission. That wonderful blouse that you purchased in the market may be embroidered with designs that inform all within range that the wearer (in this case, you) is an unwed mother of five busily looking for a husband. Only kidding, but you get the idea. An acquaintance once journeyed out on a Dakar street wearing a boubou newly acquired in the market. Little did she know that the boubous sold in the market were for tourist consumption only. They were thin and see-through, made to be worn at home and not as street clothing. As she strode through the sunlit streets clad only in her new boubou, with no slip or lining, she revealed many of her charms and an appalling lack of taste to the Senegalese, who were quick to comment.

I too have been guilty. During the superethnic seventies, I was very proud of my large collection of African trade beads that I wore on all occasions. On all occasions, that is, until a West African friend discreetly took me aside and told me that the beads were traditionally worn around the waists of young girls and that my wearing them was the equivalent of going around with a sanitary napkin proudly hanging from my neck. Well, need I say more? Know what you are wearing and what it means.

Ethnic dressing is fun. Think of the photographs of Frida Kahlo and of her delight in wearing traditional Mexican garments, or of the fun you had as a youngster dressing up in clothing from your mother's grown-up culture. It's a way to disguise yourself and yet remain yourself; to pay tribute to cultures you admire or to make a proud statement about your own ethnic roots. Take it a little at a time for starters. Go to the source yourself and bring back from vacation a piece that tempts you. The timid can begin at home with a lounging outfit. Otherwise, pair black silk evening pajamas with a smashing red silk kimono for a special evening look. Top off a fantastic white summer outfit with a twist of real or fake turquoise jewelry and a shocking pink Mexican rebozo. Enjoy the comfort of wearing a *paréo* or a *pagne* fabric wrap around the house with a shell or a T-shirt. It's easy.

Wonderful, you say, but I have a straight-arrow job and the mere word *ethnic* sends shock waves down the corridor. What do I wear? Ethnic dressing in a corporate setting demands a true sense of your own personal style. While many offices have moved away from considering gray flannel suits and blouses with pussycat bows the only acceptable office wear for female executives, some have not moved far. For most corporate women, then, the best solution remains accessorizing in a manner that speaks of who you really are. Try a bright-colored shawl that you park on the back of your chair to ward off drafts, and not incidentally to protect from terminal office drabs. Slip an embroidered Chinese silk blouse under a formal business suit. Belt your winter coat with a Navajo concha belt (a real one if you can afford the investment). A small headband of Ghanaian *kente* or a hand-painted silk scarf from Tunisia can brighten your look and your day. Almost anything will work as long as your exotic elements are selected to harmonize with your general look. If a jacket of Ghanaian *kente* is too much for you to contemplate wearing over your charcoal gray business skirt and white blouse, do as I have done and use a strip of the fabric as a belt. Try to avoid the ubiquitous one-strip priest's shawl look adopted by those who have transformed the royal fabric of the Ashanti into a cultural touchstone for many African Americans who do not know its true origin. Experiment with selected pieces and your own wardrobe, and you'll find that you don't have to look like a gypsy to enjoy ethnic dressing.

At home is the best place to get adjusted to ethnic dressing. Begin with the simplest garment—the *pagne* or sarong. Worn throughout Africa and in Southeast Asia, the *pagne* is nothing more than two and a half yards of fabric that is wrapped around the body in varying ways. In Tahiti the cloth is called a *paréo,* and the *paréo* has gone on to become the symbol of Club Mediterranée and a jet-set beach necessity. I first came across the *pagne* in Senegal, where I had purchased my first real boubou. That is to say, I had had one made by a girlfriend's tailor. Readying myself to go out for the evening, I put it on over a long slip that I had. Going out the door, I was stopped short by a "Where do you think you're going in that!" from my friend. "Out," I explained. "Oh no," was her reply, "you can't wear a boubou without a *pagne.*" So a *pagne* I wore. She instructed me how to wrap it and even gave me a piece of cord with which to attach it firmly around my waist so that it wouldn't fall down. I wore the *pagne* that evening with no mishaps, I'm proud to recall.

On subsequent trips I began to purchase *pagnes.* Formal *pagnes* are stiff fabric that is handwoven in strips or bands and then sewn together into a larger piece of cloth. Some of the best in Senegal are made by the Manjak weavers. I have two of them, one given to me in strips (the traditional manner). Heavy, handwoven formal *pagnes* are also given as symbols of wealth at weddings. My most prized *pagne* is one given to me by a girlfriend. I earned this *pagne* by being the person who introduced her to her husband.

Immediately following formal Senegalese *pagnes* in luxury and in cost are *pagnes* made from thin bands of woven fabric alternating with bands of colored cotton cloth. I have several of these, which are more comfortable to wear. They fit well under boubous for all but the most formal ceremony and can be bought in shades to harmonize or contrast with the formal boubou.

Finally, there are the *pagnes* of brightly printed cotton cloth that are worn around the house. These come in a variety of designs. In Senegal, they are sometimes decorated with batiks of fish, masks, or flowers, and come in shades of blue, brown, rose pink, and green.

Ironically, these fabrics have a long and tortuous history that combines capitalism and colonialism, and until the late seventies they had very little to do with African industry at all. The fabrics that were known in the United States as dashiki fabrics originated in the sarongs of Southeast Asia. In Bali, Singapore, and Malaysia, they're still worn today with *kebaya* tops as the national dress or sarong *kebaya.* The designs were brightly colored batiks that were hand-produced by artists. These fabrics were originally brought to the West African coast as trade items by the Dutch, with the English and others later following suit. They were liked and adopted as part of traditional dress. Indeed, in areas like Togo and Benin, these printed fabrics are still the basis for national dress. Many West African women still look for the label saying Véritable Wax Hollandais (true Dutch wax) on the selvage as a guarantee of authenticity, although now most West African countries are producing their own designs in their own mills in order to compete with the European trade. Fabric is an important item in the balance of trade, so much so that some West African countries have attempted to outlaw or highly tax European fabrics so that their own will be purchased. Whether European or African, the fabric is sold in *pagne* lengths at markets throughout Africa.

To anyone who has ever worn or used a *pagne,* they rapidly become indispensable. When traveling, I always have one or two with me—usually in my carry-on luggage, for they begin to be useful right on the plane. Folded tightly and rolled up, they are the perfect neck roll for sleeping; unfurled, they ward off the usual airplane drafts. In the hotel, they can serve as a coverlet for a quick nap or even take the place of a hideously colored bedspread. At the beach, they can serve as beach wrap or beach blanket or even beach towel, in a pinch, and when called on to attend a formal evening, they can be transformed into passable evening attire with a few strategic knots and a camisole top. Finally, there is nothing more comfortable for padding about in.

Basic Pagne Wrap

Topped by a camisole or T-shirt, this is around-the-house wear for many West African women. I even have a girlfriend from Bahia, Brazil, who knots her *pagne* firmly over a silk blouse and wears it to work with stockings and high heels.

1 pagne or 2½ yards of forty- to forty-five-inch-wide fabric, narrowly hemmed on the edges

If you're a bit larger in size, you might wish to have slightly more yardage.

Standing with your camisole or leotard top on, spread your legs slightly, as this will give you room to walk once the pagne is attached. Then, holding the fabric behind you, take one of the free ends of the long edge of the fabric in each hand. Wrap the left hand and its cloth around your waist and hold it. Then, wrap the right hand. Anchor each end, tuck the fabric ends firmly in, and verify the fit. (You may find that you don't feel secure. If not, for the first few times, feel free to cheat with a belt or piece of cord holding up the *pagne* more firmly.) Alternately, if your waist is narrow enough, you can simply knot the two long ends of the fabric. You're now dressed in your *pagne.* As you tie more and more *pagnes,* you'll begin to have a feel for exactly how you like it. Remember, if you've bound yourself at the beginning by tying it too tightly, it's not sewn—just undo it and retie it with your legs farther apart.

As you get used to working with the fabric, you'll discover that you're on the lookout for new ways to tie *pagnes.* You might even think of having a shorter one sewn out of a lightweight wool for street wear. If so, then you'll only need a thirty-six-inch-width fabric unless you are very tall.

If you fall in love with *pagnes,* as I did, you'll find that as you travel, your eye will automatically find suitable fabric. Africa reveals indigo-dyed cottons and damasks, bright traditional prints, the colorful *kitenges* and *khangas* of East Africa, and a host of woven fabrics. Southeast Asia offers block prints and ikats and a stunning array of batiks. The saris of India make superb evening *pagnes,* if you don't mind cutting them, and what could be more luxurious than a *pagne* of pure Thai silk in a brilliant color with a matching shawl? Enjoy the variety, magnificence, and beauty of the fabrics of the world.

JEWELRY

One way to ease ethnic pieces into your daily look is by wearing ethnic jewelry. Portable wealth is the name of the exotic woman's jewelry game. Anyone who has lived in turbulent times can understand why. When the going gets tough, it's good to have a little gold or silver with which to make your getaway. A friend of mine who collects ethnic jewelry once confessed that it made her feel good to know that if things got really rough, all she had to do was tuck her bijoux into a loaf of bread and head for the border. Some antique Chinese ornaments reflect this consideration; their gold weight was incised on them so that unknowing women couldn't get shortchanged by un-scrupulous moneylenders.

Abundance is another watchword for our taste in jewelry. If one is good, two are better and ten are fantastic. This goes for everything from earrings to bracelets to necklaces. Multiple ear piercings are the norm among the Peul women of Mali and Burkina Faso, while incised silver or gold bangles called *chooris* are worn by the women of Trinidad, not just those of Indian descent. Multiple ivory bracelets and armlets are a part of the dress of the married women of Rajasthan. Gold, silver, copper, brass, and bronze jewelry can also be a sign of social status, like the traditional Western wedding ring or the nose ring that Hindu brides wear through their left nostrils at traditional wedding ceremonies. Jewelry can be a talisman guaranteed to protect the wearer from harm or evil, like the Moroccan hand of Fatima or the Turkish evil-eye beads. It can even be a sign of a religious covenant, like the tiny glass-bead necklaces worn by Brazilian and Cuban practitioners of Can-domblé and Santeria.

The Chinese have worn jade for millennia. The well-to-do wore beads of jade, coral, agate, or pearl in the summer and switched to ivory and cedar ones in the winter. Jade is still talismanic for many Chinese. "Jade," Confu-cius said, "shines like benevolence; it is strong and dependable like wisdom; its edges are sharp but do not cut, like justice, and like truth, it does not hide its flaws." I once received a gift of jade from a dear Chinese friend who has since journeyed to the land of the ancestors. The gift was accompanied by a note saying that jade is the cement of friendship. I looked at the beautiful jade fish that seemed alive in my hand. It was truly a talisman to keep. Even today, walking down the streets of Hong Kong, Taiwan, or Singapore, it is wonderful to look at the wrists of wizened Chinese grandmothers and teenagers alike and notice that all have a simple circlet of jade around them. Tradition has it that you should not purchase jade for yourself, so hint strongly to someone that you'd love a piece. You won't regret it.

Brazilians also have their talismanic jewelry. Many of them wear a clenched-fist charm called a *figa*. Figas come in all sizes, from the massive life-sized wooden ones that decorate the trays of Bahian women who sell street food, to tiny gold ones that are small enough to fit on a watchband. *Figas* are thought to be protective. Like jade, they cannot be purchased by the individual who is going to wear them; they must be received as gifts.

In the 1970s and early 1980s, I was the proud owner of an armful of an-tique ivory bracelets that had been given to me in various parts of West

Africa. They were so much a part of me that they virtually became my trademark, and people who didn't recognize my face remembered the bracelets. On a trip to India, by the side of a Rajasthan road, members of the group and I were leaning over a wall looking down at a group of washerwomen as they went about their daily chores. Soon, the women became agitated and kept pointing at our group. I finally realized that they were pointing to me. Then, the penny finally dropped. They were admiring my armful of ivory which, although from Africa, looked for all the world like their very own ivory bracelets. We began to signal each other with gestures and giggles and only parted after smiles and waves. Some pieces and some things are international.

Silver pieces also abound in the exotic world. They range from heavy Berber fibulae that women use to hold their cloaks together, to the intricately filigreed *keronsang* that the Nonya women of Singapore use to fasten their *kebayas* or blouses. Native American jewelry from the Southwest is some of the most collectible silver jewelry around. Navajo squash-blossom necklaces tell a history of world design. When the Spanish conquistadores arrived in the Southwest, their horses' bridles were hung with talismanic emblems, including the crescent moon, which the Spaniards had appropriated from the Moors who had occupied their country for hundreds of years. The Navajo, in turn, borrowed the symbol from the Spaniards and called it the *naja*. It hangs at the bottom of every squash-blossom necklace. Traditionally, these necklaces were worn by young girls, for the squash blossoms that decorate the necklace symbolize fertility. Concha belts, from the same area, are another classic and look perfect with everything from jeans to black cashmere. These one-of-a-kind masterpieces of fine craftsmanship are striking fashion pieces, but they're expensive. Remember, you're purchasing pieces with a tradition, not just a mass-produced item signed with a designer's name.

Semiprecious-stone necklaces are still relatively reasonable and can be obtained at mineral stores and jewelry shops. Think of malachite or coral, amber or turquoise. The latter three can go up in price if you want the rarer types. Coral jewelry is highly valued in Nigeria and Brazil. In Martinique, menopausal women wore coral jewelry, which was thought to protect from hot flashes, or garnet, which was said to be good for the eyesight. In fact, the code of Creole jewelry was such that women in mourning even wore mourning jewelry of jet. (No gold was permitted.)

Gold, though, is the standard for the most luxurious ethnic jewelry. It's an expensive but worthwhile investment. Senegal, in West Africa, is noted for the filigree work of its jewelers, who spin spider's webs of gold into necklaces and earrings. In Ghana, farther south, they make more massive pieces, using thin sheets of pure gold. Pre-Columbian pieces from South America—go hyperventilate on the windows of the gold museum in Lima—are extraordinary. Jewelers offer replicas in gold or vermeil and bronze, depending on your pocketbook. As with all pieces of gold worldwide, items called gold may be as low as ten-karat gold (in parts of the English-speaking world) or as high as twenty-two-karat or even twenty-four-karat pure gold (in Turkey and parts of India). Prices will vary accordingly. Be sure that you know the karat before you buy, and always buy from reputable jewelers.

In Martinique and Guadeloupe in the French-speaking Caribbean, while the rich Creole landowners' wives wore pieces from Europe, the mulatto elite and women ranging in social status from slaves and courtesans to market women and wet nurses—indeed, all but the very, very poor—wore gold jewelry acquired a bit at a time. Restricted by sumptuary laws that legislated matters of dress for mulatto and slave women, they still stamped their originality on the jewelry of the region. Slave mistresses wore the *chaine forçat,* a gold-link chain that signaled their "special" status as the master's favorite. Wet nurses traditionally raised two generations of a family and wore the jewelry that they received from them on special holidays. Their pride and joy was an accumulation of tiny striated beads called *choux,* which they wore in a single long strand wrapped around their necks many times. They also had baby teeth and hair mounted on tiny trembling brooches called *tremblants.* Market women and others wore what they could afford and what they could save for, including the daily *créoles* or hoop earrings, which took four to six months to pay for. Provocative temptresses called *matadores* were always bedecked in the gold jewelry that remains today one of the glories of the islands: necklaces like the *collier choux* and the *chaine forçat.* They also wore the *grain d'or* necklace of gold beads, which was created because black women were not allowed to wear pearls, as well as other pieces of jewelry that took their inspiration from the world around them. Earrings called dahlias, wasps' nests, custard apples, and *tété négresse* or black ladies' breasts (they're conical and pointy) are all part of the traditional Creole jewelry box.

There are no rings in the jewelry of the French-speaking Caribbean. Women of color have always been conscious of their hands, perhaps because they labored with them. Why are there no traditional rings? The answer is logical: because the women worked with their hands!

Jewelry is worn daily, but the jewelry coffers are truly flung open on occasions like christenings and weddings and, in Guadeloupe, at the annual Feast of the Women Cooks in August. I had to have a pair of *tété négresse* earrings for the name alone. When I purchased them at a jeweler's in Martinique, I was astonished by how light and delicate they were. They joined my collection of antique pieces from Brazil, Senegal, and India. My mother, who makes beautiful eighteen- and twenty-two-karat gold pieces, wears only button earrings and the occasional necklace. Select what works with your own personal style. If you get "hooked," try jewelry auctions, thrift shops, consignment shops, yard sales, and even your grandmother's jewelry box (with her permission, naturally). You never know what you'll find.

Not all ethnic jewelry is expensive. Try wearing colorful ropes of glass-bead necklaces on a white dress, as the Bahianas of Brazil do. String them yourself out of your favorite colors, or purchase them already strung and heap them on.

In West Africa, young girls wear ropes of small glass beads around their waists under their clothing. In Senegal, these beads are called *ferre* and are considered very private and personal. The reason is that when the girl has reached puberty, these beads are a sign of her womanhood and are something for only her and her lover to know about. The memory of the rhythmic clicking of the beads when the young woman walks is thought to remind her lover of her and of the pleasures of the bed. In bed, the friction of the beads is said to add an extra something special to lovemaking.

Senegalese Waist Beads

Enough brightly colored small glass beads to fit loosely around your waist

Elastic string

String the beads on thin elastic thread in any design you wish. The strings should be long enough to slip on over your head and to encircle your waist loosely, but not long enough to fall off. Wear the waist beads under summer shifts and with your bikini, or wear them in the privacy of your boudoir. They'll set off the warm color of summer skin perfectly. And who knows, they may add a *je ne sais quoi senegalaise* to your lovemaking.

(If you are slightly hirsute in those regions, you may find that the elastic string snags and is painful. In that case, use regular string and add ribbons to the ends of it so that you can tie the beads loosely around your waist.)

The women of Senegal and Mali have honed adornment of the body to a fine art. Some of them don't stop with waist beads but add the extra dimension of scent. Strings of myrrh beads are mixed with strings of beads prepared from natural tree gums and made fragrant with a personalized scent. This takes a bit more doing but is a fun project to attempt when you have some time.

Malian Scented Waist Beads

3 tablespoons gum arabic

1 tablespoon sweet almond oil

A few drops of your favorite essential perfume oil or musk or amber essential oil

Mix the ingredients together in a small bowl until they form a thick paste. Using your fingers, roll the mixture into small beads. (Think kindergarten!) Pierce the beads with a large needle so that they can be easily strung. Allow the beads to harden overnight. Then string as directed in previous instructions for Senegalese

Waist Beads. You can add powdered spices to the mixture or a bit of your own individualized incense.

In Mali, these scented beads are worn with several strands of small myrrh beads. They are stored in tightly sealed jars filled with incense or potpourri, which keeps the scent fresh. When a woman wears these beads, she's surrounded by a veil of scent that is uniquely her own. She's also wearing a unique and very personal form of ethnic jewelry.

Even feet get into the jewelry picture. My friend Nicole, who is Belgian but lives in Dakar, Senegal, was the first to tell me of her toe ring. Her husband was a Toucouleur.

Toucouleur Toe Ring

Toucouleur women in Senegal and Mali wear toe rings to placate the genies of the feet and to give them steady footing. You can wear your toe ring for sure footing, too, or simply for the fun of it. Toucouleur toe rings are simple knobbed bands of copper, silver, or gold that are worn just below the toenail around the first joint of the second toe. You can have one made to order for a pittance at a jeweler's, or you can choose any simple adjustable ring and place it on your toe. Choose one without snaggy projections, so that it will fit into sandals and even under closed shoes and stockings if necessary. Nicole wears hers all the time, whether dressed in European couture or in a bathing suit and *paréo*. Once you've found the right one, clamp it around your toe and head off.

FRAGRANCE

A final touch, one without which no exotic woman would think of setting foot out of her house, is a veil of perfume. After all, as part of the legacy of Avicenna (the Persian who invented the distillation process), perfume is a part of the exotic woman's birthright. Rose waters, orange-blossom waters, musky oils, grainy dry perfumes, light floral fragrances, and all manner of incenses are used. Fragrant roots, aromatic gums, flowers, herbs, and spices are mixed to create potent incenses that perfume not only the women, but also their clothing, their undergarments, and their bed linen. These final personalized touches are part of the total sensory experience that transforms women of color into the birds of paradise, flamingos, and peacocks of our world.

Perfume has been around longer that we imagine. The word itself goes back only to the Romans and comes from the Latin *per fumare*, meaning "through smoke." That's exactly how the first fragrances wafted through the air. Before the Romans named it, though, the Egyptians burned blends of spices, herbs, and odorous gums in large braziers to scent their rooms. Cleopatra is said to have used as her individual fragrance a blend of sandalwood, winter's bark, orrisroot, patchouli leaves, myrrh, woodrose, and olibanum. This was burned in great bowls in her living quarters and thought to promote peacefulness, serenity, and, of course, romance.

This form of incense was not the Egyptians' only use of scent. Their main use of aromatics was for embalming the bodies of their departed ones, but aside from that, their world must have truly been a scented paradise. Henna flowers and other fragrances perfumed the sails of royal barges, signaling their arrival long before they could be seen. Aristocrats carried small balls of aromatic resin with them to perfume the air. At dinner parties, guests were offered cones of scented tallow, which they would place on their heads. As the evening progressed, the cones would melt in the increasing heat, dripping scent all over the individual and perfuming the room.

The ancient Hebrews also appreciated scent, and the Bible is full of references to frankincense and myrrh. In fact, one of the world's oldest cosmetic recipes is one for anointing oil found in the Bible.

> *Moreover the Lord spake unto Moses, saying*
> *Take thou also unto thee principal*
>   *spices, of pure myrrh five hundred*
>   *shekels, and of sweet cinnamon half so*
>   *much, even two hundred and fifty shekels,*
>   *and of sweet calamus two hundred and fifty*
>   *shekels*
> *And of cassia five hundred shekels after the*
>   *shekel of the sanctuary, and of olive oil*
>   *and hin*

And thou shalt make it an oil of holy ointment
an ointment compound after the art of the
apothecary: it shall be a holy anointing oil.
EXODUS 30:22-25

The Babylonians, too, loved scent, and by edict of King Hammurabi everyone had to bathe and perfume frequently. The Arab world was truly a scented garden, with musk and rose the predominant perfumes. If roses scented the Arab world, jasmine is the undisputed scent of the Far East. In India, fans, screens, furniture, and almost everything imaginable are carved from fragrant sandalwood, which was also used in facial cosmetics and burned as an incense. In *ayurveda,* or Indian holistic medicine, it is considered relaxing, an antidepressant, and even an aphrodisiac. Other favored Indian fragrances were vetiver and patchouli. The former was woven into screens that were used to mask the heat of the day and into fans that were moistened and used to circulate the torpid air. Patchouli was used as a natural moth repellent. Indeed, the original cashmere shawls that were sent to European markets were pungent with patchouli, so much so that when Europeans began to manufacture their own shawls, they scented them with patchouli as a marketing ploy.

In the colonial Caribbean, the heady odors of musk and *khus khus* (or vetiver) were popular. The Creole empress Joséphine Bonaparte was particularly partial to musk—even today, the walls of her bedroom at Malmaison retain the fragrance. She was also fond of violet perfume.

Slaves in the United States had little time for perfuming themselves. However, the scents of clean clothes and fresh flowers went a long way. Occasionally, a timid finger was dipped into the vanilla extract of the kitchen and applied behind ears as a fragrance. Native Americans used fragrant grasses and herbs to perfume themselves.

The scents of women of color are as personalized and as special as their dress. They range from the light Florida waters that members of New World Yoruba religions use to purify themselves, to the powerfully heady *gongo,* a powdered perfume from Senegal that is said to have potent aphrodisiac properties.

⚜

Caribbean Bay Rum

Bay rum, like most classic colognes, is unisex and can be used by men and women alike. Keep a bottle of it in the refrigerator during the summer; a cooling splash is positively invigorating.

A 2½-cup bottle or jar

1¼ cups 60 percent alcohol (you may use inexpensive vodka instead)

½ teaspoon oil of bay

3 drops oil of orange

1 tablespoon dark Jamaican rum

¾ cup water

Place the alcohol or vodka in the bottle. Add the essential oils and allow them to dissolve in the alcohol. Add the rum and the water, close the bottle tightly, and shake it gently to mix the ingredients thoroughly. Let the bay rum "mature" for a week. After a week, decant it into a fancy bottle for presentation. You may want to add a bay leaf in the bottle for decoration. Shake well before using.

If you bottle the bay rum in fancy cut-glass bottles or in antique perfume bottles, it makes a lovely gift.

—— ❀ ——

Moroccan Orange-Flower Water

Orange-flower water is used just about everywhere in Morocco. It's used cosmetically and in cooking, and after meals it is sprinkled on guests' hands from chased-silver sprinklers. Try using some in finger bowls at your next formal dinner party. Sprinkle some on your guests' hands after a meal, or simply soak small washcloths in it and present them to your guests after the next party with finger-licking-good food.

    4 drops oil of orange
    4 drops oil of bergamot
    ½ cup 60 percent alcohol (vodka may be substituted)
    1 cup water

Dissolve the oils in the alcohol. Then add the water to the alcohol, mix thoroughly, and allow to stand overnight. It's ready to use. Unless you use essential oils that are pure enough to consume internally, this orange-flower water is not for cooking use.

—— ❀ ——

Florida Water

Florida water is a light, refreshing cologne that is both inexpensive and widely available in the Hispanic and African American communities, where it is believed to have special spiritual properties. For many Santeros and Santeras who follow the Yoruba religion of West Africa as it is maintained in Cuba, Florida water is also considered a purifying agent. Not a believer? Don't worry; you can simply enjoy the light fragrance.

1 teaspoon lavender oil
1½ teaspoons oil of bergamot
½ teaspoon lemon oil
2 drops musk oil
2 drops jasmine oil
2 drops rose oil
2 cups 60 percent alcohol
2 tablespoons rose water

You may wish to change the proportions of the oils slightly so that the final Florida water will bear your individual imprint.

Dissolve the oils in the alcohol in a small jar. Add the rose water to the alcohol and oil mixture and close tightly. Mix well by shaking gently; then let sit overnight. The following day, decant into fancy jars. You may want to keep one in the refrigerator for a cooling splash.

Vanilla essence has been used as a perfume ingredient for years. It is the only orchid used in perfumery and one of the world's most expensive spices. I can smell its distinctive fragrance in such favorites as Guerlain's Shalimar. In times when Shalimar was out of the question, and in fact no colognes were available, women turned to what was at hand and discovered that vanilla essence used alone gave a soft warm scent that was both subtle and alluring. It's a fragrance that's as close as a trip to the pantry and one that's guaranteed to make you smell good enough to eat.

Vanilla Dip Perfume

1 bottle vanilla extract

Simply dab a tiny bit behind each ear when desired.

The fragrances of the exotic world of women of color are myriad. Which one appeals to you? Try a different one for each of your changing moods. The following are some essential oils you may wish to try.

Amber. This rich oriental scent reminds some of musk. It seems to conjure up thoughts of harems and sultrily beautiful women. It is thought to be healing, to strengthen the aura, and to enhance telepathic powers.

Bergamot. This essential oil is produced from the fruit of bergamot oranges, which grow mainly in Italy. It has a lush orange fragrance with an undertone of spice. It is used by some for protection.

Cedarwood. The Queen of Sheba's mouth "dropped like a honeycomb and the scent of her garments was the scent of Lebanon." The fresh, clean, woodsy scent of cedar has been prized for millennia. Think of cedar chests and cedar closets. The ancient Egyptians used cedar for embalming. Assyrian women ground cedarwood with cypress and frankincense and mixed it with water to make a paste for softening their skin. The fragrance of this wood, which the ancient Egyptians thought to be eternal, is said to promote wisdom.

Clove. Zanzibar is the isle of cloves, and its scented breezes waft the spicy fragrance of its clove trees to all visitors. The pungent oil reminds some of baked hams and kitchens.

Frangipani. The rare oil is all too often only a blend of essences. True frangipani, a lush, exotic floral fragrance, is reputed to be good for those doing psychic work. It comes from the *Plumeria rubra* plant, which is native to the Philippines but grows in parts of the Caribbean, Africa, and the South Seas. Tahitians use this plant, which is also known as red jasmine, to weave crowns called *tiare*.

Frankincense. Also called olibanum, and one of the gifts of the biblical wise men, this essence is still precious. It has one of the longest histories of any scent. Native to the Middle East, Africa, and India, this gum resin was used by the ancient Egyptians. Its religious significance spans millennia, and it is still used today in much traditional church incense. For many, therefore, its pungent, distinctive smell is most often associated with old cathedrals.

Gardenia. In ancient China, the gardenia was the flower of November. In the West, it's a symbol of hidden love. It is said to be protective, calming, and soothing. The gardenia's fragrance is sweetly floral. If you use it, think of Billie Holiday, but don't sing the blues.

Jasmine. Originally from India and Persia, jasmine has a long history. In India, Kama, a god of love and a cousin of the Western Cupid, was said to scent his love arrows with jasmine flowers. In China, jasmine was used to throw on floors, to flavor and scent tea, and to adorn the hair of young women. It was also used to cleanse sickrooms. On the streets of Hammamet, Tunisia, today, it is possible to purchase a sprig of jasmine to scent the night with a sweet floral fragrance that is at the same time delicate and heady.

Lotus. Associated with Egyptian magical rites, the lotus flower represents the highest in spiritual concepts. Its sweet, heavy scent is thought to attract good fortune and love. It is also considered a sacred flower in the Far East, where it occasionally represents spiritual enlightenment.

Musk. When the prophet Mohammed describes paradise in the Holy Quran, he mentions that the ground is flour mixed with musk and saffron and that "the houris were made pure musk." The natural fragrance comes from a sex gland of the male musk deer, which gives its life to produce this essence. For that reason, most of the musk used today is synthetic. True musk is found only in the finest of perfumes. The fragrance is considered an aphrodisiac by much of the world. The musk oils of the 1960s and 1970s pale in comparison with the odor of true musk. An indispensable substance in perfumery, true musk is one of the most expensive of all perfume elements.

Myrrh. Mentioned in the Ebers Papyrus, one of the longest and most famous documents relating to the medical practices of ancient Egypt, myrrh has a history that goes back almost four thousand years. The myrrh tree is a native of Somalia, Ethiopia, the Sudan, and parts of southern Arabia. Its resinous gum was burned as incense in Egypt; it was prized by the Queen of Sheba; and it too was one of the gifts of the magi to the Christ child in the Christian Bible. Like frankincense, it is pungent and heavy.

Patchouli. Anyone who lived through the sixties knows the scent of patchouli. Ironically, the "sixties" could be the 1960s or the 1860s, for the fragrance enjoyed popularity in the same decade of two centuries. In the 1860s, it was popular because patchouli leaves were used to pack cashmere shawls. In the 1960s, the heavy, woody scent signaled rebellion against more traditional values. Patchouli originated in the Philippines and Indonesia, but will always be associated with the Indian subcontinent in the minds of the West. The leaves are also used in some religious ceremonies to bring harmony.

Rose. This is it, the queen of all essences. In the Middle East, it is the fragrant symbol of the prophet Mohammed; it is said that when he ascended to heaven, the first rose sprang from a few droplets of his sweat. It is likely that the rose originated in Persia, but it and its fragrance have taken over the world. Preserved roses have been found in Egyptian tombs. In India, one of Vishnu's wives was found in a rose. In Morocco, rose water is used to flavor tea and even some desserts. *Urgujja,* a salve used by Arabian women, contains attar of roses along with jasmine, sandalwood, and aloe wood. Legend has it that attar of roses was discovered in a most romantic way. In ancient Persia, during an extravagant celebration of a royal wedding, the palace canals and fountains were filled with rose water and rose petals. After the festivities, it was noticed that an oily layer had formed that had a delicate, but intense fragrance of roses—thus attar of roses was born. The fragrant floral bouquet of roses is still one of the world's most expensive perfume essences, and one of the most popular.

Sandalwood. What roses are for much of the Arab world, sandalwood is for the Indian subcontinent. Mentioned as early as the fifth century B.C., the tree has been cultivated in India for millennia. It is used there for building, and shavings are burned as a purifying incense. The wealthy dead even have logs of sandalwood added to their funeral pyres, and it turns up in numerous beauty preparations. Sandalwood's distinctive woody yet spicy fragrance perfumes everything from fans to furniture to the carved screens hiding zenana quarters. The scent lingers for years, giving unopened drawers and stored linens the fragrance of a ghostly presence.

Vetiver. This woodsy-fresh fragrance smells pleasantly of damp green underbrush and conjures up images of both India and the tropics. In India, the aromatic roots are used to scent clothing, and mats woven from it are hung at windows, dampened with water, and used to protect from the heat of the day. In Martinique and Haiti, fans woven from vetiver are moistened to produce similar effects. The fragrance is also used in Candomblé houses of Salvador da Bahia, Brazil, to scent and purify.

Ylang-ylang. Potently floral with sweet undertones, this "flower of flowers" comes from the South Pacific. The women of Tahiti mix it with their coconut oil as a body rub and hair oil.

The list of essential oils is seemingly endless. These are simply some of the ones most in use in the exotic world. They can be found in some health-food stores and at herb shops and new-age stores. They can also be ordered by mail from the purveyors listed in appendix A. Remember that there are natural essential oils and synthetic ones. The natural ones are more costly by far. They are also much purer; a few drops will do, and they are so pure that they cannot be used without being diluted in an oil like a sweet almond oil or in a perfume diluent. Try blending a scent that is uniquely yours or simply layering on several different oils for a personal fragrance. It's the final touch to a truly well-adorned body.

☙

Chapter 7

SHARING WOMAN-SECRETS

Just Between Us

"Shhh. . . . It's a secret."

W OMEN ARE ALL BOUND TOGETHER in an international secret sorority sealed by an initiatory blood oath. We love secrets and we keep the secrets of the world. To some, secrets may appear selfish, but there's no denying the thrill of having personal knowledge of something special. It may go back to the time that you actually bought the first holiday gift for your parents that they didn't know about, or to thoughts of love locked away in a diary or whispered over the telephone to your very best friend. Then there are lovers' secrets of special spots, unique feelings, and tender words. And, of course, there are beauty secrets.

In the Western world, women do not have as many occasions to share beauty secrets as they do in other societies. In West Africa, women talk while preparing communal meals. Advice flies while yams are being pounded in mortars and fish is being grilled over *feu malgache*. While sitting in *hammams*, Moroccan women enjoy a sense of feminine community that is becoming rare in our world. They sit scrubbing away at each other's backs and feet, and tales of traditional remedies and recipes for beauty secrets flow as openly as the perspiration released by the purifying steam. In Mexico, a late-afternoon siesta may bring no rest, but instead turn into a small, adult version of a pajama party, with women discussing herbal baths, makeup suggestions, and tales of how they worked when last used. Coming-of-age ceremonies for women in Native American societies acquaint girls with the secrets of womanhood and women's links to the earth and the cycles of continuity. In the sultry warmth of a Caribbean night in rural Haiti or Jamaica, you're sure to find women sitting out in the yards or courtyards of their homes in a traditional pose. One is sitting at the other's feet getting her hair braided, and both are busy discussing all manner of secrets—from new lovers to dress patterns to what to do to get that man who lives down the road who is so-o-o fine. Secrets are shared, advice is given, and the continuity of traditional beauty is maintained during these impromptu sessions.

If you know a woman from the exotic world, you have only to begin to ask her what to do for menstrual cramps or problems with pregnancy to be regaled with a wealth of solutions. She'll be able to tell you of at least one solution she remembers her grandmother or great-aunt or best friend's mother using with much success. She'll be able to regale you with tales of aphrodisiacs, both proven and dubious, and will quite possibly leave you laughing uproariously at their effects. Depending on her depth of knowledge, she may be able to tell you of teas to brew to induce abortion and others that will help promote conception. She may even take you over to meet her grandmother or aunt for a session with her.

I was privileged in Martinique to have a friend treat me to one such session with her aunt, a venerable lady seventy-eight years young. Madame Renée lives on the southern end of Martinique right alongside the entrance to a huge Club Mediterranée. Entering her front gates, though, time seems to drop off and you're transported to another era, an earlier Martinique. Her small wooden home seemed sacred, and indeed was surrounded by lush vegetation and fenced-in areas full of the gentle cooing of doves. It was raining, so we headed into the house. "It used to be my family's vacation house," she says, settling into her rocking chair and taking my measure, trying to see if and why I'm interested in her and in the traditional ways of Martinique.

Her eyes close and she decides I'm okay; I've already decided I adore her. Such a long distance to discover I'm at home. Madame Renée, whose face reminds me of relatives, is a one-woman walking encyclopedia of the herbal lore of Martinique. Moreover, she is witty and wise, with a wicked sense of humor. We speak for hours about the old ways: of herbal baths and healing cures, of how to bathe babies and how to stop pimples. Her words are punctuated by strident cries of *"Ah bon!"* (Oh good!) from her African gray parrot that sits on the floor beside her chair. From time to time, Madame Renée hops up and darts out to the garden to pluck a leaf from this bush and a berry from that one to make sure that I am clear on what she's discussing. Our conversation lasts well beyond the allotted time, and we part only with regret because of other engagements. I hope to return to Martinique to spend more time sitting at the feet of Madame Renée.

Madame Renée and women like her all around the world are our memory. They're willing to share their secrets; all we have to do is listen. They hold keys to solving problems of headaches, menstrual cramps, constipation, and colds. They know how to eat well for beautiful complexions and how to transform a wallflower into a vamp. They know how to catch and keep a man and how to keep their own personhood in the process. They've got something to say about everything from sexual tricks to coquetry. They know the secrets of the world.

COLDS

Conversations about special secrets always seem to begin with someone saying, "Why didn't you tell me you had that? My grandmother had the perfect cure. In fact, it works so well, I still use it." And then she goes on. June, a colleague and friend of mine from Guyana, said just that one day as I was sniffling my way through a long stretch of work with what was obviously a wicked summer cold. She said one word, "Aloe," and then went on.

June's Cold Remedy

When I first heard of June's cold remedy, finding aloe was the hardest part of the cure. Today, though, I live in a neighborhood where the vegetable shops bristle with produce from the American South and from the Caribbean, and blades of fresh aloe are available virtually year-round.

1 fresh aloe blade	Sugar to taste

Slit the spiny leaf of this cactuslike plant with a knife and remove the jelly. Place it in a small glass bowl. Sweeten the jelly slightly with sugar. Brown cane sugar would be most authentic, but whatever type you have is fine. Take a teaspoonful two or three times daily for the cold.

June's cold remedy is just one use for the marvelously versatile aloe plant. The most common uses are external. Aloe is used to soothe burns ranging from sunburn to small kitchen burns. The leaf is again split. This time, though, the jelly from the leaf is smeared on the burned area. It works wonders on minor burns, and I know many people who keep a small aloe plant on the kitchen windowsill for just that reason.

The Chippewa made a sweetened tea of wild onion and drank it to rid themselves of some of the symptoms of colds. They also chopped up cowslip roots and boiled them in water. This potion was said to induce perspiration and loosen phlegm. In South Carolina's low country, sea myrtle and sea-eye ox are brewed as teas and taken for colds.

In the Bahamas, catnip is steeped in boiling water and then taken as a tea for colds. Alternately, a mixture of honey, lemons, and finely minced onion is prepared and allowed to steep. The resulting syrup is taken a teaspoonful at a time three times a day. Fever is cured by steeping fresh peppermint in hot water and drinking it as a tea until the fever subsides. They also use watermelon to cure chills and fever. The seeds are steeped in boiling water and drunk as a tea until the fever breaks.

Hiccups

Colds and fever we all get; hiccups, though, are a plague in my family and dogged my late father's path. Whenever he was ill, they would appear to add their insult to the injury of illness. Once, when he was in the hospital, needing treatment for another ailment, along they came. They rang out loud and clear and, as anyone who has ever suffered from hiccups knows, made his life miserable. Finally, a nurse wise in traditional African American ways stopped them with a simple trick. No, it's not blowing into a paper bag or holding your breath. It's easier than any of those. And what's more, it works.

Hoagy's Hiccup Cure

Don't think about it. Just try this remedy the next time you or anyone you know gets hiccups.

1 small piece of brown paper about half an inch square

Moisten the paper with a dab of water and stick it to the middle of the sufferer's forehead. Leave it there until the hiccups subside. I don't know why this works; I can only speculate that the concentration goes from the hiccups to the dab of paper and therefore the cycle is broken. I can say, though, that my father's hiccups, which had been known to achieve three-day longevity, disappeared every time that Hoagy tried this. If you know a hiccup sufferer, give it a shot—it certainly couldn't hurt.

Most of us who lead fast-paced lives sometimes have days when waking up is just a prelude to feeling tired. If this happens to you, try doing what the Brazilians do: get an extra jolt of energy with a bit of *guarana. Guarana,* an Amazonian plant, has three times the caffeine of coffee. Brazilians buy it pulverized into a powder and take some with their morning fruit juice to get them hopping (literally). The taste is something like chocolate, and Brazilians swear that *guarana* not only gives you more energy, it also makes you think more clearly and therefore function better. Remember, though, because of its high caffeine content, a little bit goes a long way. *Guarana* in powdered form can be found in many health-food stores.

Maté, the herbal tealike beverage that is the drink of choice of the Brazilian and Argentine gauchos, is another way to start your day with a bang. It too is loaded with caffeine and can also be found at health-food stores. If you are caffeine-sensitive, you should leave *guarana* and maté alone or you'll be spending a night or two searching the ceiling for spots.

While Brazilians swear by *guarana* and maté, Chinese and, increasingly, many other people around the world swear by ginseng. Ginseng has been in Asia since before 3000 B.C. Sometimes known as "man root" because it can assume near-human shapes while growing, ginseng is reputed to be everything from an aphrodisiac to a tonic. It has become a remedy for almost every ill imaginable. It can be used in facial masques and bath herb mixtures, taken internally as a tonic, and used in other ways too numerous to mention. In China, though, they know one thing about ginseng that we seem not to have understood: too much is not good for you.

CRAMPS

Cramps can be the bane of many women's existence, returning with clockwork regularity. Some women manage to escape them entirely. Others, though, are so bothered that they take time off from their jobs and take to their beds until the pain subsides. Women around the world have, for generations, used a number of teas and tisanes to relieve the pain of cramps. When asked, they're only too ready to give a suffering "sister" some advice.

Beatriz's Oregano Tea

Beatriz gave me this recipe one day while we were in the market in Mexico City. She was picking up some extra dried oregano to brew a pot of tea for a co-worker who was having painful cramps.

1 tablespoon dried oregano
1 cup boiling water

Place the oregano in a tea ball or in a small square of clean cheese-cloth. Pour the boiling water over the oregano and allow it to steep for five minutes. Remove the tea ball and drink the tea while it is hot. You can also just allow the oregano to steep and then strain the hot tea into another cup.

In Jamaica, several years back, I discovered that while many folk were certainly smoking marijuana, the old folk simply used it as one of their traditional herbs and brewed a tea from it, a tea that they served with milk and sugar in true British fashion. I was amazed.

Granny's Not-Quite-Legal Ganja Tea

Needless to say, this recipe, like Alice B.'s brownies, is just for your edification and not for your use. But it's a surefire cramp cure.

1 to 2 teaspoons of ganja (depending on the strength)
1 cup boiling water
Milk and sugar to taste

Pour the boiling water over the ganja and allow it to steep for ten to fifteen minutes. Don't spend your time inhaling the vapors. Strain out the herb, reheat the tea if necessary, add the milk and sugar, and drink while hot. Your cramps will no longer pain you. You may still have them . . . but you won't care.

When I moved from Manhattan into a neighborhood that is half African American and half Caribbean American several years back, I discovered that a whole world of traditional remedies was lurking at my greengrocer, just waiting for me. One day I came across Jamaican 151-proof Wray and Nephew rum. When I asked a Jamaican girlfriend about it, she told me that many Jamaican women consider the white overproof rum to be a necessity as a traditional Jamaican cure for cramps.

Maria's Wonder Waters

It's simple and it works. The principle is much the same as with Granny's Not-Quite-Legal Ganja Tea: the cramps may still be there, but you no longer care.

¼ cup Wray and Nephew 151-proof white rum

2 ice cubes

Splash of water

Twist of lemon

Place the rum and ice in your favorite glass. Add the splash of water and the twist of lemon. Voilà, you have a cramp-relieving cocktail. It's strong and one will usually do the trick, but if necessary you may repeat judiciously. And don't let anyone call you an alcoholic—this is for medicinal purposes only!

All cures for cramps from the exotic world are not alcoholic or illegal. June, my Guyanese best buddy and true "sister," gave me this one from her country.

June's Cramp Cure

Although June has an American doctorate and is a college professor, when she wants true remedies, she returns to her Guyanese roots and comes up with gems like this spicy-gingery cramp-relieving tea.

2 teaspoons powdered ginger

5 whole cloves

1 cup water

Place the ginger, cloves, and water in a small nonreactive saucepan and bring them to a boil. Lower the heat and allow to simmer for five minutes. Strain and drink while hot.

Ginger, which is among other things an antiflatulent and digestive aid, is used by Chinese women for cramp relief.

Chinese Ginger Tea

This tea uses freshly scraped gingerroot. If you go to a Chinese neighborhood where you can get tender young gingerroots, the tea will be more fragrant.

1 cup boiling water

1 tablespoon freshly scraped gingerroot

Bring the water to a boil in a small saucepan. Place the freshly scraped gingerroot in a small nonreactive bowl and pour the water over it. Allow the root to steep for at least five minutes; then strain the liquid and drink as a tea. You'll find that this tangy, bitey tea will help cure some of the pain of cramps. The Chinese also have a ginger syrup that is available in wonderful small pots. A teaspoon or so of it in a cup of hot water will do the trick as well.

I'm always on the lookout for soothing, calming nighttime beverages. Many years ago, I found out about chamomile tea. I'd actually known about chamomile tea ever since I'd read *The Tale of Peter Rabbit* as a child. I knew that it was a great tisane to take after dinner or at bedtime, but I never connected it with cramps until Wilma, a southern friend of mine, informed me that she'd been drinking it for years. I headed off to a health-food store and bought several ounces of the tiny yellow flowers and have been dispensing them to cramp-plagued friends ever since.

Wilma's Chamomile Cramp Tea

    1 tablespoon chamomile flowers
    1 mug boiling water
    2 teaspoons honey, or to taste
    ¼ lemon

Place the chamomile flowers in a small bowl and pour the boiling water over them. Allow them to steep for five to seven minutes. Then strain out the blossoms, pour the tea into a mug, and add the honey and a squeeze of the lemon. Drink the chamomile tea while it's hot. You'll be surprised at the taste. I still can't understand why Peter Rabbit didn't like it.

Native American women have remedies for cramps as well. Many of the traditional ones involved the herb pennyroyal. Pennyroyal is the strongest member of the mint family; it is wonderful in potpourris and sachets for repelling insects. The Kiowa women used to brew a pennyroyal tea to relieve cramps. Pennyroyal in large doses can be toxic, however, so I've replaced it with peppermint, which is perfectly safe.

Kiowa Tea

1 tablespoon fresh peppermint leaves
½ tablespoon fresh dandelion blossoms

Boil the mint leaves and the dandelion blossoms together for seven to ten minutes. Then strain out the herbs and drink the liquid as a tea. If you cannot find dandelion blossoms, the peppermint will work by itself.

Raspberry Leaf Cramp Tea

Raspberry leaf tea is another tried-and-true cramp reliever. You can find dried raspberry leaves at most herb shops.

1 cup boiling water
1 tablespoon red raspberry leaves

Pour the water over the raspberry leaves and allow them to infuse for ten minutes. Then strain out the leaves and drink the tea while it's hot. If you really want extra relief, couple this tea with vitamins B, D, E, and calcium.

DOUCHING

To douche or not to douche is a question for which there is not yet a definitive medical answer. Many exotic women, though, have devised special-purpose douches that are reputed to do everything from tighten the vagina to aid in conception to catch a man. For centuries, African American women in the rural South used alum douches to temporarily tighten their vaginas. A Mexican friend told me that friends of hers take herbal baths prepared from *romero macho* (male rosemary), which is said to shrink and tighten vaginal muscles. She then added a personal story to demonstrate a surprise effect of this bath.

Although the friend and her husband had been married for several years and had never used contraception, she had not conceived. She had begun to take baths of *romero macho* to tighten herself up when suddenly, she was pregnant. Amazed, she asked a friend who was wise in the ways of plants and was told, "But of course, baths in *romero macho* are also taken to aid conception." She was surprised to say the least, but now she is the proud mother of a fat little baby boy. Her attempts at solving one problem ultimately cured two.

A simpler way to douche, and one that is unlikely to increase your chance of pregnancy, is one from the Dominican Republic. There, and throughout the Caribbean, those who go to beaches with the local folk will notice that the older women don't really go into the water but tend to sit at the water's edge, letting the waves gently lap at their bodies. These women are no fools. They're getting double benefits: first, they're digging their feet into the smooth-packed sand at the water's edge and smoothing the callouses and dead skin off their feet; second, they're enjoying a public, yet oh-so-private personal cleansing courtesy of the salt water, which acts as a personal douche.

A traditional African American douche is a tried-and-true favorite that is even being recommended by gynecologists as one of the best. It's as simple as vinegar and water.

Old-Time Vinegar-and-Water Douche

¼ cup distilled white vinegar

3 cups water

Mix the vinegar and water together in a douche bag and proceed as you would normally. This mixture is particularly effective because it closely approximates the slightly acid pH of the vaginal area.

Followers of the Yoruba religion turn to the goddess Oṣun for advice on matters sexual. A priestess friend of mine suggests this man-attracting douche and predicts great results.

Oṣun Douche

1 tablespoon honey   4 cups water

Mix the honey and water thoroughly in a douche bag and proceed as you would normally.

If you really don't want to try an Oşun douche, but you like the idea behind it, try a trick from Marlene, a Brazilian friend of mine. When you're going on a manhunt, to a party, or on a special date, wear bright yellow underpants. Yellow is Oşun's favorite color, and some Brazilian women feel that she will keep a special eye on them if they signal their devotion to her. I must have looked skeptical, because my friend then added that on the days leading up to New Year's Eve in Rio de Janeiro, it's impossible to find a pair of yellow underpants in any shop.

PREGNANCY

Eating is taken particularly seriously when a woman is pregnant. In many cultures, there are strict regulations as to what she should and should not eat. In China, some of the rules go back as far as the thirteenth century A.D., during the Yuan dynasty, when they were written down by four of the emperor's doctors in the *Yinshan Chengyao*. Pregnant women were told:

- Eat no rabbit as it makes the child dumb and encourages a split lip.
- Eat no lamb as it gives the child many diseases.
- Eat no chicken testicles and dried fish as it gives the child boils.
- Do not eat duck and mulberries together as they cause reverse birth.
- Do not eat sparrow meat and alcohol together as it results in the offspring being shameless and oversexed.

Turtle meat was thought to give the child a short neck. Donkey meat was thought to delay births, and mule meat was said to give a difficult labor (perhaps because then the child became as stubborn as a mule about making an entrance into this world).

The Carib Indians, who gave their name to the Caribbean region, also thought that what you ate contributed to who you were. For them, this dictum extended beyond the period of pregnancy. They believed that eating turtle meat or pork made people stupid. Pork, which originally came from

Europe, had the extra onus of giving people beady eyes. Crabmeat was never eaten before a long voyage, because it was thought to cause storms at sea.

For the Chinese, though, foods were not the only items to come into play in this way of thinking. There were also animals and other objects that pregnant women were supposed to contemplate. Gazing at dogs and eagles was thought to make a child strong and healthy. Looking at carp and peacocks would produce a clever child, and contemplating pearls and jade would result in a beautiful child.

A contemporary Chinese woman informed me that even today Chinese women are very selective about their food intake while pregnant. They avoid peppery food, as it is considered bad for the complexion of the child as well as for their own. They do not eat snake for fear of giving the baby snakelike skin. They will eat things that are good for the baby and look at beautiful pictures in order to produce a beautiful child.

The African American world is not as specific about do's and don'ts, but pregnant women are constantly cautioned not to look at unpleasant sights.

Pregnancy inevitably leads to either births or miscarriages or abortions, and the exotic world has a number of aids for each. Abortion, though, is not common in the world of exotic women. When circumstances necessitate it, however, it is practiced. In some cases, the difference between labor aids and abortifacients is only in the dosage. The Zuni of western New Mexico brewed a tea from flatspine ragweed that was used to promote menstruation. The Alabama and Kosati brewed a tea from the roots of the cotton plant that was originally used to ease labor. It was found, though, that in high doses the same teas would induce abortion.

African American slaves who did not wish to bring children into a life of enslavement used the roots of the same cotton plant that was the reason for the enslavement of many to induce abortion. The root stimulates the uterus and causes contractions.

Pregnancy is also a time when the women of the exotic world take particular care of their bodies. In parts of West Africa, shea butter or *karité,* the miracle natural emollient, is called into play. Pregnant women give their expanding bodies a daily gentle rub with the vegetable butter. Many of my friends there have assured me that this daily routine prevents stretch marks. In Jamaica, the same daily massage is done, but with coconut oil instead of shea butter.

When the time of birth arrives, the exotic world provides so many differing aids for the discomfort of childbirth that a simple listing alone would take up another volume. They include everything from belly dancing to black-pepper tea. Many of the teas that are used to relieve menstrual cramps do double duty easing childbirth pains.

My Gypsy friend, Morocco, an instructor in belly dancing and a specialist in the dances of North Africa and the Middle East, explained to me that one of the possible origins of belly dancing lies in exercises that women were given to ease the difficulties of childbirth. By strengthening the lower abdomen with these exercises, the women were able to deliver with greater ease. Watching the sensuous, sinuous movements of Morocco's expert dancing, it's easy to believe.

Not all remedies, though, require that you move your feet. In the Bahamas, at the first signs of labor, midwives brew a tea of a handful of fresh thyme steeped in boiling water. The tea is allowed to cool and then is consumed by the cupful each hour until delivery. They also brew a tea from black pepper that is cracked and then steeped in boiling water. The tea, which is taken warm, is consumed at four-hour intervals until delivery. In Martinique, Madame Renée tells me that women cook okra in water and drink the liquid from the pot in the hours prior to giving birth. Cherokee women were given a tea prepared from the inner bark of the wild blackcherry plant during the early stages of labor to relieve pain and act as a sedative. On the other side of the world, in Mongolia, the beginning of labor is the time to take a tea prepared from juniper leaves and ground gingerroot.

Nursing

Nursing mothers throughout the exotic world soothe tender nipples with creams made from coconut oil, *karité,* sesame oil, and other emollients. Arab women eat borage while nursing; it is said to increase their milk supply. In parts of the African Atlantic world, women know that when the time has come for the child to stop nursing, a touch of bitter aloes on the nipples will usually do the trick.

Teas and Herbal Drinks

Women of the exotic world have consumed teas and herbal drinks for centuries, not only to ease the pain of childbirth, but also for everything from gastric problems to nervous disorders. I first learned about tisanes or herb teas in France while there as a student. I noticed that whereas many Americans like to finish their meal with a cup of coffee, it is common in parts of Europe to finish up with a tisane. The choice is wide, and almost all restaurants can comply with a request. There are chamomile, a perfect nighttime drink; elderflower, a stimulant; peppermint to settle the stomach; nettle for rheumatism; and linden blossom, which is perfect for relieving headaches.

I was doubly surprised on my first trip to West Africa when at the end of one of my first meals on the continent, a friend appeared with a steaming pot of lemongrass tea. It smelled familiar, but it took me a while to figure out what it was. It was citronella, the same citronella that we had burned when I was a child to keep away pesky mosquitoes during summer barbecues. As a tea, it was aromatic and seemed to smell slightly of lemon. It was a perfect ending to a perfect meal, and I went off to sleep like the proverbial baby.

It was only on a later trip that I discovered the quintessential West African tea—*kinkeliba.* This is an herb tea that is taken for medicinal and for pleasurable purposes from Senegal to Benin. It grows wild and now has become so popular that it is packaged in tea bags commercially in Senegal. Some of the best that I ever had, I picked for a colleague from New York who was naming her art gallery Kinkeliba House in honor of the plant and its properties. I found it growing wild in the grassy area surrounding the Portuguese fort at Ouidah, in what was then called Dahomey. When it was brewed into a tea, it was soothing and calming.

I seem to ferret out the tea that I need in my life when it is helpful. I drink lavender tea to raise my spirits. Chamomile helps put me to sleep. Rosemary helps with headaches and colds. Borage works as a pick-me-up after a rough day, and verbena helps me to calm down. I brew them all to a basic recipe.

Herbal Teas

1 tablespoon dried herb	1 cup boiling water

Pour the boiling water over the herb in a china or porcelain cup. Allow the tea to infuse, and drink it hot. If you are preparing tea in a pot for several people, allow an extra tablespoon of dried herbs "for the pot." Don't forget to sweeten the tea with honey. You'll get more benefits than you can imagine.

APHRODISIACS

In the Yoruba religion, honey is one of Oṣun's secrets, and she uses her honey (taken literally by some and figuratively by others to mean her female sexuality) to captivate men. Honey is a potent addition to any aphrodisiac that comes out of this tradition. This is fascinating when it is remembered that honey is a natural spermicide as well as a natural antibacterial. You don't have to be a Yoruba to know about Oṣun's power. I was astonished when a very proper New Orleans matron recounted how, in the wilder days of her youth, she had come home from a party "knee-walking drunk" and scraped her knees. "I immediately put honey on them to heal them," she added. I don't remember the rest of the story because I was so transfixed by her reference to the medicinal use of honey. When I asked, she, in turn, was astonished; she'd thought that everyone knew that honey was perfect for healing small scratches, cuts, and abrasions. Her ancestors might have learned the healing trick from women from Martinique who, when they eat honey, always dab a bit on their faces because it softens the skin and makes it smooth.

Honey is not the only aphrodisiac in the exotic world. Many foods and substances, from Spanish fly to rhinoceros horn, are reputed to have aphrodisiac qualities. The poor, nearsighted rhinoceros has been hunted practically to extinction because the Chinese consider its horn to have potent aphrodisiac qualities. Other aphrodisiacs are more easily available and do not cause the extinction of an animal. One evening at dinner in Dakar, Senegal, I noticed that my Senegalese "brother" was busily chewing on radishes as though they were going out of season. His munching and crunching was accompanied by what seemed to be ribald comments in Wolof from his male friends. When I asked what the jokes were about, I was told that in Senegal radishes are considered aphrodisiacs. Remember that when you make your next salad.

On Saturday night in Port of Spain, Trinidad, any visitor can see men lined up around the vendors' stalls on the Queen's Park Savannah. "What are they doing?" is the question posed by many an unwary tourist. The usual answer is, They're getting their ration of mangrove oysters, served with hot sauce, before their Saturday night date. Most are satisfied with that explanation. Not I. I pursued the subject until I got the real answer. In Trinidad, as in many other parts of the world, oysters are considered an aphrodisiac. The men were simply stoking up their furnaces in preparation for what they hoped would be an eventful night ahead. In Nassau, in the Bahamas, those crossing the bridge to Paradise Island may notice that the conch vendors' stands under the bridge seem to have a clientele consisting almost completely of Bahamian men, along with the occasional tourist. Guess why? The conch salad and cracked conch that they sell are reputed to have great aphrodisiac qualities.

In Senegal and Mali, women prepare and use a dry, powdered perfume that has had astonishing effects on many a man. It's called *gongo*. Prepared from dried rhizomes that are pounded into a powder and then perfumed with aromatic oils and spices, *gongo* has a particular musky smell that harmonizes well with any perfume and indeed with any woman's own personal scent. Traditional women wear small cloth sachets of *gongo* on their waist beads, and more modern ones tuck a sachet in their bras. Their body heat helps the *gongo* to release its musky aroma.

I first read about *gongo* in an amusing short story about a man who was so entranced by the fragrance of *gongo* that he spent all his fortune, sacrificing it and ultimately himself, in order to purchase more and more of the substance for his wife. Intrigued by the idea of a perfume that could have such results, I began my quest for *gongo* in Dakar, Senegal. I badgered friends, who by now thought I was nuts anyhow, haunted the local Sandaga and Tilene markets, and generally made a nuisance of myself until I found the name of a woman who made *gongo*. I immediately commandeered a taxicab and gave the driver her address.

By the time I arrived, she had already prepared a bottle of *gongo* for me. In the traditional no-waste ideology of the Third World, my *gongo* came in a large serum bottle that was being recycled from some hospital. I asked the price and was quoted a high one that indicated the *gongo*'s value to her. I paid gladly, as I'd almost given up hope of finding any. I had been back in the taxi, clutching my serum bottle of *gongo* wrapped in a length of fabric, no longer than a few minutes when the driver's nose began to twitch. He gave me a curious glance in the rearview mirror and then asked me in French what I had stopped to do. I hesitantly explained my *gongo* excursion and watched as a smile gradually crept across his face from one ear to the other. "*Gongo,*" he exclaimed, complete with rather frightening cries of delight. "*Gongo!* An American who knows about *gongo*. Who would have thought it!" I rode back to the hotel with the grinning driver shaking his head.

Gongo, I found out when I finally got to examine closely the contents of my serum bottle, is a grainy powder with a musky-spicy aroma to it. A pinch of grains tucked into a bra will leave its scent for a day and slightly irritate the skin in a not unpleasant way. This slight irritation is perceived as stimulating by many, and couples who can afford it have been known to rub *gongo* over each other while making love. The slight irritation and the fragrance add another dimension to lovemaking. I gave small pillboxes filled with *gongo* to friends for years, and it made many converts. I also discovered, on subsequent trips, that there is no definitive *gongo*. Each woman prepares it according to her own recipe—some are more pungent, others more citrusy, others almost pure musk. I did learn, though, that the fragrance of *gongo* lasts for quite a long time. I still have some of that first serum bottleful tucked away in a drawer and each time I open the drawer, I get a whiff of *gongo* and the memories of my cab ride. Then, too, my *gongo* adventures (over which we'll draw the veil of discretion) waft back to haunt.

Unfortunately, *gongo* is not available in the United States, and I have not yet been able to determine the botanical names for the rhizomes from which it is prepared, or a reasonable substitute. However, if you have an adventurous friend who is going to Dakar, ask her to look for *gongo*. You'll love the story of the reaction of the Senegalese, and the *gongo* itself is certainly worth a try.

Find a special perfume that works for you and your lover and use it only when making love. The silent looks of complicity that you'll share each time one of you gets a whiff of the fragrance will add another dimension to your lovemaking. Let it just be one of our little secrets.

Chapter 8

LIFE ENHANCERS

Home Is Where the Heart Is

TRADITIONAL

THE QUALITY OF YOUR LIFE shows on your face. Your happiness reflects itself back at the world through the twin mirrors of your eyes. Your lightness of step evokes the approach you have to the path that has been created for you and by you in this world. These are obvious truisms. Most of us can instantly recall a friend who, no matter what blessings life bestowed upon her, was never quite happy. We have all met people who have the ability to turn diamonds into dust, to snatch defeat from the jaws of victory, and to just plain put a damper on anything. Don't get me wrong, my name is not Pollyanna. However, I truly believe that your attitude, outlook, and environment can do a great deal to keep your inside harmony radiating outward as beauty. Where and how you live influence how you feel.

Look around you. The Romans said, "A healthy mind in a healthy body." We know that. That's why so many of us are out there exercising ourselves into good health. But what about the environment in which that mind and body must exist? Is your harmony reflected in the space that is your own? Whether it's one-third of a dorm room, a cramped studio apartment, a loft, house, mansion, or lean-to, your home reflects you. It's your sanctuary from the world, and for many of us it's our workplace as well. Let it reflect you.

Ever since I had my own room, and that's been as far back as I can remember, I've been influenced by my surroundings. I'm so influenced that when I travel, I take a few small mementos of home with me to place around and transform my hotel room into a temporary home. I always have pictures of loved ones in a small silver frame, my *pagne,* which can do double duty as a bedspread, neck pillow, or body wrap, and a small stuffed animal for company. Once, in Dakar, my friend Elaine walked into my hotel room and said, "Jessica, I'd know your hotel room no matter where you are in the world; you always personalize it." I've been known to place bedspreads in the closet for the duration of my stay and move furniture around, much to the dismay of chambermaids. I get cranky in an environment in which I'm not comfortable.

PURIFICATION OF SPACE

It's not about money or space; it's about creating your world with what you have. Whatever space you have, when you begin to occupy it, the first thing that you should do is purify it. The first apartment I ever lived in was brand-new and I was the first tenant. Once I signed the lease, I stopped at a neighborhood florist and bought a small bunch of eucalyptus leaves and a vase. The dried eucalyptus leaves scented the air and also signaled that I had taken possession of the space. When I moved to my second apartment, I did the same thing. My house, though, had been owned by others before my tenancy, and so the old ammonia and water came out and I scrubbed down the entire house. Ammonia is considered a neutralizer of evil spirits in the Yoruba religion.

When I moved into my house, even stronger measures were called for. This was beyond ammonia. My house, a handyman's special, had been lived in by generations of folk who had cared not one whit for its beautiful oak stairway, its incised slate fireplaces, and its magnificent proportions. The wooden front door had been painted a horrific Day-Glo electric blue, and the crown moldings of the dining room were papered over in aluminum foil. Everything was in need of attention: you could almost feel that the house itself was unhappy. Ayo, one of my priestess friends, suggested a New World Yoruba remedy. "Burn some asafetida," she said. "Just wait until you are sure that you're leaving the house. Find a stable incense burner that you can hold in your hands and walk with. Start at the top of the house—the attic, if you can get there. Then light the incense and walk with it through each and every room of your house. Walk from top to bottom, heading toward the front door. When you arrive at the front door, leave the incense burner in a basin of sand, so that there is no danger of fire; leave the house and let the asafetida burn out. When you return the next time, the house will be purified. Follow this with a scenting with your favorite incense."

I followed Ayo's instructions, with one addition. When I told my friend June, from Guyana, what I was doing, she said, "In Guyana, when we purify something, we use white lavender." I couldn't find white lavender, but my second scenting was done with purple lavender, which I burned on charcoal. When I returned to my home after this two-pronged attack, it was almost as if the house reached out to embrace me, saying thank you. Okay, I know it sounds nuts. Perhaps it's all in your mind, but the point is, you can harm no one and you have indeed claimed your space as your own.

Societies much older than our own have used incense to communicate with the spirits for centuries. In pre-Colombian Mexico, the Aztecs used copal, a tree resin, in their religious ceremonies. Various groups of Native American peoples often begin their ceremonies with smudges from many plants—most commonly, tobacco mixed with other plants—to purify the air and create a sacred space. In Taiwan, fragrant coils of incense and joss sticks are visual manifestations of prayer wafting its way toward the heavens. In Salvador da Bahia, Brazil, negativity is cleaned out of many Candomblé believers' homes every Saturday by burning a purifying incense prepared from branches of thyme mixed with frankincense and myrrh that is purchased in the Mercado Santa Bárbara. This is the method that I used. Try your own.

Home Purifying

1 basin filled with sand or nonflammable kitty litter

2 small pastilles burning charcoal for incense

1 stable incense burner

2 ounces asafetida (or the papery outsides of a mixture of onions and garlic)

2 ounces lavender blossoms

Be sure to select an incense burner that you can hold in your hands while it is burning. Some get too hot, so choose carefully!

After you have emptied the space that is to become your home of all the previous owner's items and cleaned it thoroughly, purify it. Before beginning, place the basin filled with kitty litter behind the entrance door; you'll need it later. Then head to the top of the house or the back of the apartment or loft. Place one of the charcoal pastilles in the incense burner and light it according to directions. When it is hot enough to burn red-orange, drop a few pieces of the asafetida onto it. The asafetida will have a pungent smell that is slightly like burning onion or garlic. Then, holding the incense burner in your hands and thinking positive thoughts about your new space, walk slowly through each room of your house from top to bottom. Don't forget closets and basements, and even the attic, if you can get there. When you arrive at the front door, place the incense burner firmly in the sand so that it will not tip over and start a fire. Then leave the house for a few hours.

When you return, place the second charcoal pastille in the incense burner and return again to the top of the house or the back of the apartment. This time, sprinkle lavender blossoms on the burning charcoal to perfume your home-to-be with pleasant smells. Once again, walk toward the front door. When you're finished this time, extinguish the incense and go on about your business.

Brazilian Purifying Incense

This is not quite the same incense that they sell in the Mercado Santa Bárbara in Salvador da Bahia, Brazil, but it will do the same job. Use it periodically to "clean" your environment.

1 ounce dried thyme	¼ ounce frankincense
½ ounce dried rosemary	⅛ ounce myrrh

Mix all of the ingredients together and burn over charcoal.

Native Americans use grasses and plants to purify their space in much the same way. The four primary plants that they use are sweetgrass, tobacco, sagebrush, and cedar. They are sometimes referred to as the Spirit Keeper plants. Sweetgrass is woven into thick braids and used as a smudge by some Native Americans. It is considered to represent the energy of the earth. Among some groups, the long fibers of sweetgrass are called "the hair of the mother," to signify its connection to the earth, mother of all plants. Tobacco, one of the most sacred Native American plants, is thought to bring clarity to those who use it appropriately. For many Native American groups, smoking tobacco is calling upon the spirits for help. Sagebrush (not culinary sage, with which it is sometimes confused and which is another frequent ingredient in Native American smudges) helps bring change. The final of the four Spirit Keeper plants is cedar, which is purifying.

Native American Purifying Smudge

A combination of sweetgrass, tobacco, sagebrush, and cedar

1 earthenware bowl or incense burner

1 large pheasant or turkey feather

Select the combination of plants that represents the properties you wish to invoke. Then place them together in the bowl and light them. Begin at the rear of your space and walk through it, wafting the smoke through the atmosphere. Use the feather to keep the plants smoldering.

Note: The tobacco that is in cigarettes will not work for this process; it is too full of adulterants to have all its properties. Use tobacco that you have purchased from an herbalist or the best cigar that you can afford.

Interestingly, in the Cuban version of the Yoruba religion, tobacco is also used as a smudge. This time, though, the tobacco is in the form of cigars that are used for their smoke, which is blown backwards through their tips by putting the fiery ends in the mouth. This is definitely an acquired skill, but it will also work to purify your space. If you cannot smoke the cigar backwards, simply treat it with respect as a sacred tool and smoke it normally. Purchase the most expensive cigar that you can afford and use it only for that purpose.

DECORATION

Once you have established yourself in your space, then you must make it your own. It's your sanctuary from the outside world, so decorate it with talismans of your own life. Surround yourself with photographs of friends and heirlooms from family. Everything from beach glass picked up on a vacation to a length of fabric that was wrapped around a gift you once received should find a place. Ascetic or accumulator, the style is up to you. Now, I guess you've figured out that I'm not a decorating minimalist—my friends call me the grand acquisitor. But even if you are a minimalist, select and enjoy the items that are a part of what makes you, you. Here are some suggestions from friends' homes around the world.

I write cookbooks, and so I spend a lot of time in the fancy decorator-designed kitchens of my colleagues. One of my favorite kitchens in the world, though, was one that belonged to my friend Khadijah. An American who has ended up transplanted in Paris after a personal odyssey that took her to much of West Africa, Khadijah is a woman of majestic African size. Khadijah loves to eat, yet for years she amazingly didn't know how to cook. I remember one summer in the open market in the Cocody suburb of Abidjan, Ivory Coast, instructing her how to prepare fresh string beans. She was amazed at how simple it was. When we caught up with one another again several years later, she had mastered cooking with a vengeance. She, in fact, hosted many a Sunday brunch for members of the African American community in Paris and had equipped the kitchen of her rented Parisian apartment with a caterer's *batterie de cuisine*. Abundance was the watchword. Baskets from around the globe hung from the rafters above her stove. Earthenware casseroles and cooking pots tumbled over one another in her pantry, and enough glassware to serve an army battalion was lined up neatly on her shelves. Seasonal fruits and vegetables were piled up on the counters, and the whole kitchen seemed to glow with the energy and warmth of someone who loves to cook and who loves to entertain.

Khadijah had created the perfect environment for herself and her love for food and entertaining. The rest of her home was minimalist, but in her kitchen the abundance with which she greets her guests showed joyously.

Kitchens are the central rooms of more than one home in the exotic world. In African American homes, best friends enter through the kitchen door, and sometimes it feels as though you can't get them out of the kitchen into the rest of the house. This makes it the perfect room for displaying small collections and cherished objects. My friend Lurita collects salt and pepper shakers, and her collection has grown enough to have tumbled over into the living room as well. At a roadside stand in Guadeloupe, I once saw an array of bottles of flavored rums lined up simply in the sunlight. It's a perfect way to treat a kitchen window with a less-than-wonderful urban view.

Baskets of seasonal produce are hallmarks of markets in exotic countries around the world. Place the ingredients for your dinner salad in a basket for color, or purchase a string of garlic or a *ristra* of chiles. Containers of copper, brass, and clay, calabashes, gourds, and baskets are found in kitchens throughout the exotic world. They are a perfect way to bring the world of exotic women into your own space.

Bedrooms are personal havens from the world, a place where we rest and recoup. Here the women of the exotic world offer many tricks—from how to scent the rooms to how to dress the bed—and our decorating styles are as numerous as we are. Think of the shoji screens, tatami mats, and futons of the rustic inns called *roykans* in Japan, or the lavishly painted walls of the zenana quarters at the palace in Udaipur, India, where the very walls seem to exude sandalwood and it is impossible not to think of nautch dancers and sensuous nights. Think also of nights under Bedouin tents, or of sleeping in thatched rondavels where each animal's sound is magnified manyfold by the surrounding silence.

I've always loved bedrooms, and I still remember the joy of being able to sleep on a camp bed, or better yet a pallet on the floor, when spending the night at my grandmother's house as a child. Just nestling into her home-made quilts while dozing at the side of her bed was my childhood dream of perfect bliss.

Today, my favorite bedroom is in Jamaica, where my friend Norma has a bed-and-breakfast near Montego Bay. My room, when I'm there, is a hedo-nist's hideaway. Located at the water's edge, the room is not lavish. In fact, it's rather sparsely furnished. A white-wicker furniture grouping invites you to sit and read, while an enormous bed covered with vast white mosquito netting in-vites you to sleep and dream. Through the window opposite the bed, there's nothing but the Caribbean Sea and Montego Bay. At night, it's heavenly to sit and watch the lights twinkle across the bay.

Bathrooms are as close as most of us will get to spas. My friend in Sene-gal, Carrie, had the bathroom of my dreams. A large mosaic soaking tub set on a pedestal dominated the room. Dakar's markets had yielded an array of unguents and incenses, and local perfumeries had provided Parisian bath oils, bubbles, and perfumes. That was fantastic enough, but the best thing about Carrie's bathroom was that, through the window, you could hear the sound of the ocean. The waves of the ocean lulled and soothed you while the small currents of the soaking tub washed away all aches, dirt, and troubles.

We're not all as fortunate as Khadijah to have Paris's many markets at our doorstep, or as Norma to have Montego Bay's lights for nighttime illumi-nation and decoration, or as Carrie to have the ocean beyond her bath. My own bedroom looks out on the exceedingly urban view of a brick wall. The dorm room that I had in college was so small that it was called the broom closet by one and all. Both were transformed into warm, inviting spaces: per-sonal havens where peace was found.

The world of the senses is a primary concern in the environmental world of exotic women. After all, they live in areas of the world where sight, smell, touch, and hearing are tantalized daily with colors, aromas, textures, and sounds that the rest of us can only dream about.

Think of the colors of the fruits arrayed in the open Feira São Joaquim market in Bahia, Brazil—the new-leaf greens of *xuxu,* the bright reds and or-anges of chiles, the deep purples of eggplant. Remember the multiple hues of a sunset over Hawaii that seemed to contain the entire spectrum of reds and yellows, or the deep shades of violet, turquoise, and indigo in a display of Kanchipuram saris in southern India. Think of the colors of Ghanaian *kente* and Thai silk, of Ecuadoran weaving and Zairean *kassai* velvet. All these colors are but a fraction of the color possibilities from the exotic world. Anyone who has ever seen a Senegalese woman glide down a Dakar street knows about the excitement of dazzling color combinations. What about brilliant yellow with deep purple? Or shocking pink and aqua? Not all the colors of the exotic world are brilliant: think of the muted pinks, ochers, and roses of the American Southwest and the multiple tones of beige and brown found in most deserts.

Color may take over a room and transform it into a rug seller's stall in the Grand Bazaar of Istanbul, or it may be a subtle highlight, like a single cactus flower blooming in the Mojave. The point is that your environment should be a feast for the eyes. *Plaisir des yeux,* the French say—a pleasure for the eyes.

No matter how beautiful your home is, no one will want to enter if it doesn't smell inviting. Here again, women of color have a multiplicity of ideas. After you've purified your space, don't put the incense burner in the closet and forget it. Use it! Your home doesn't have to smell of the heady, heavy perfumes that we think of as oriental. Use your incense burner to burn a few lavender flowers. Once while visiting a friend in California on a cool night, I was thrilled to notice that she took a few embers from the fireplace into the fireplace shovel, sprinkled on a handful of lavender blossoms, and walked through the living room giving one and all a fragrant lift.

Homes in West Africa are perfumed as well. When you walk through a doorway there, you are greeted with a warm, enveloping wave of scent. For many women, this scent is their personal incense, perfumed with their own blend of fragrances. It's called *thiouraye. Thiouraye* in Senegal is simply incense. To blend their own, the women go to the market for a dab of this and a handful of that and then return home to pound it in a mortar until it is well pulverized. They finish the mixture with additions of aromatic gums and perfume essences. The finished whole is kept in a tightly sealed jar and is sprinkled from time to time with the woman's favorite perfume. Some Senegalese grandes dames "water" their *thiouraye* with Chanel No. 5, First from Van Cleef and Arpels, Shalimar, and other fine French perfumes. The result is a scented blending of East and West that is magnificent when the *thiouraye* is burned over charcoal on cool nights.

Ever curious, I asked my friend Thiane to help me make some *thiouraye* in Senegal. We headed off to Sandaga market for the necessary items. Our first stop was to buy a pound or so of small rhizomes called *djeguidje,* which form the basis of most Senegalese *thiouraye.* Then we bought flower blossoms and other items to add. Finally, we went off to find a stall that sold small bottles of various perfume oils. The tiny blue and amber bottles were decorated with pictures of oriental minarets and harem women. All things gathered, we returned to Thiane's home to begin making the *thiouraye.*

In her sandy courtyard, Thiane dragged out a huge mortar and two pestles. She handed me one of the pestles and we got to work. This was more difficult than it seemed. While I could pound in the mortar, I couldn't keep the rhythm that would allow my friend with the second pestle to pound as well, and our pestles kept banging together. Finally, she finished pounding it on her own. When the pounding was complete, she placed the now powdered mixture into a screw-top glass jar, added some dried herbs and flowers, and finally the pungent oils that we had purchased. "When you get back to the hotel," Thiane instructed me, "pour a bit of your perfume over the *thiouraye* to give it your scent. Then keep it for a few weeks to allow it to mellow before you use it." I poured and waited, and when I finally used the *thiouraye,* back in New York, it was wonderful. The fragrance of the herbs, roots, and perfume oils blended perfectly with a hint of something that was my summer perfume. You can't make Thiane's *thiouraye,* but you can make a facsimile version using already-powdered ingredients.

Thiouraye

3 parts powdered frankincense

2 parts powdered orrisroot

1 part powdered cloves

1 part powdered sandalwood

1 part powdered patchouli leaves

A few drops of bergamot oil

A few drops of your favorite "oriental" scent

Place the powdered ingredients in a small bowl, stirring them with your hands to make sure they are well mixed. Then pour them into a glass jar that can be tightly sealed, add the oils, and stir until the mixture becomes a thick paste. Seal the jar and put it aside for two weeks. Open it occasionally to sprinkle the mixture with a few drops of your favorite perfume or eau de toilette. (The more powerful the form of fragrance you use, the more you will smell it through the *thiouraye.*)

When ready to use, light a charcoal pastille, allow it to get hot, then put a small dab of the *thiouraye* on it and enjoy your own incense. If you are lucky enough to live in a home with a fireplace, you can burn the *thiouraye* on the embers from a dying fire. You can even sprinkle a bit of it on a hot, dry, cast-iron skillet and allow it to perfume your air.

Ersatz Thiouraye

Many of us are simply not going to do the work that's necessary even for a *thiouraye* facsimile. This, then, is a simple way to prepare a *thiouraye,* one that requires nothing more than some unscented incense-type sticks and your favorite mixture of essential oils, or bath oil.

24 unscented incense-type sticks
1 shallow pan large enough to hold the incense sticks
2 tablespoons or so of your favorite essential oil mixture

Place the unscented incense sticks in the pan and drizzle the essential oils over them, making sure that each stick is well coated. Cover the pan with plastic wrap. Allow the sticks to sit for a few days, turning them occasionally, until they have completely absorbed the oils. Drain off any excess and allow them to dry. This may take a few days. Then wrap them tightly in aluminum foil. When ready to perfume your home, simply light one of the incense sticks and let your personal fragrance waft through your home.

Home Scenter

Home scenting doesn't have to be a craft project. Your favorite essential oil or bath oil can also perfume your home. It's as simple as placing a drop of fragrance on a cold lightbulb. (The lightbulb must be cold or it may break.) As the lightbulb heats up, the fragrance will begin to evaporate and you'll be soothed by an aromatic veil of scent.

If all else fails, don't forget those incense sticks that you can purchase almost anywhere. Select a simple floral fragrance like lavender or rose or an oriental blend. You can even personalize them with a few drops of an essential oil.

Incense, though, is not the only way that the atmosphere can be perfumed. At Christmastime, my mother sends a spicy fragrance throughout our home by dropping a handful of cloves into a pot of boiling water. In summer, a pot of fresh mint or other herbs growing in a kitchen window will be useful for cooking and also will bring the smells of the season indoors.

Blankets, linens, clothing, and lingerie can also be scented with sachets or bundles of spices and herbs. In Martinique, moist pods of fresh vanilla are pressed between sheets of silk paper and then placed between bed linens and inside pillowcases. A friend whispered to me that to have truly fragrant vanilla, you should soak it briefly in aged rum, scrape it with a pin, and place it on a cloth to dry in the sun. Some folk in Martinique believe that the scent of vanilla is an aphrodisiac. Also in the Caribbean, women tie a few bunches of vetiver roots with a bright satin ribbon and place them in their drawers. Patchouli is a natural moth repellent. It was used to protect the original cashmere shawls on their journey from India to Europe. Instead of using mothballs in your closet, try placing a few patchouli leaves in a piece of tulle and attaching it to the clothes rod. In parts of India, patchouli leaves and vetiver roots are used in mattresses and pillows to suppress the scent of perspiration. Try making yourself a small scented pillow. All you need is two small handkerchiefs.

Scented Pillow

>2 equal-sized handkerchiefs
>   Several ounces of your own mixture of herbs and spices
>   Thread to match the handkerchiefs

For a really fancy pillow, select handkerchiefs with embroidered designs. If you cannot find handkerchiefs that you like, simply cut two small squares or rectangles of fabric. Place the fabric pieces or handkerchiefs together with the right sides facing and sew around the edges, leaving a small hole for filling. Turn right side out and iron flat. Then fill the pillow with your own mixture of herbs and flowers. Fill the pillow with sandalwood and patchouli for scent, or lavender and pennyroyal for soothing, or hops and lemon balm for sleep. When the pillow is plump, fold the remaining edges of the opening together and stitch it closed with small, neat stitches. Scented pillows make wonderful holiday gifts.

Sachets are yet another way in which exotic women scent their clothing. Sachets can be made from almost anything, from tiny quilt squares perfumed with vanilla and orange peel, bringing the scent of the kitchen to your tea towels and tablecloths, to a crochet round lined with muslin and filled with lavender or patchouli. You can use any of your own favorite herbs and spices. This mixture I named for my Indian friend Shoba, whose home always has a wonderful hint of sandalwood in the air.

⚜

Shoba's Sandalwood Sachet

½ cup powdered sandalwood

¼ cup ground cinnamon

¼ cup ground orrisroot

1 tablespoon ground cloves

5 drops rose essential oil

5 drops lavender essential oil

5 drops sandalwood essential oil

Place all the ingredients together in a medium-sized glass bowl. Using your hands, or a wooden spoon, stir the powders together with the oils until they are well mixed. Allow the mixture to dry overnight in a tightly covered container. Prepare small cloth bags from your favorite fabric. (See the directions for preparing bags for the scented pillows and then reduce them to a size that works for you.) When the ingredients are dry, spoon them into your sachets and sew up the final openings in the bags. Place the sachets in your lingerie drawers and in your linen closet between the sheets.

Shoba's sachet calls forth the scent of India with powdered ingredients. This one, which I named for my other Indian friend, Shika, uses dry ingredients to the same effect.

Shika's Sachet

1 cup rose petals (the most fragrant you can find)

¾ cup vetiver roots

½ cup patchouli leaves

¼ cup mace

5 drops orrisroot oil

Mix the dry ingredients together and allow them to stand for one hour. Add the orrisroot oil, mixing it well with the dry ingredients. Place the mixture in a tightly closed container and allow it to "mature" for one week, opening the container from time to time to turn the ingredients and make sure that they remain well mixed. When the mixture is ready, spoon it into small cloth bags and sew the final openings closed. These bags will bring scent to your dresser drawers, closets, shoes, suitcases—wherever you stuff them.

Too tired to make your own sachets? Don't have the raw ingredients? You can still bring some fragrance to your home with nothing more than a section of perfumer's blotter and your favorite perfume or essential oil. The perfumer's blotter will hold scent much as the old store samples did.

While sight and scent play primary roles in the life environment of exotic women, the other senses come into play as well. Touch is important in the world of exotic women, and textures take on new meaning. Theirs is a world of nubby silks and heavy handwoven Haitian cottons, of rough raffia mats and baskets woven of intricate coils of sea grasses. In decorating your home, take a hint from the wide variety of natural elements available in the exotic world. Think of brass, copper, wooden, and calabash containers for everything from your mail to your knitting. Think of baskets, baskets, and more baskets, and of fabrics made from natural fibers ranging from silk to wool. Juxtapose rough and smooth, shiny and matte, and notice how your eyes begin to revel in the variety of pattern and texture. Sound is also important: try to eliminate the jangles of everyday urban life. A discreetly placed wind chime, a string of bells inside a doorway, a muted telephone, and a pleasant doorbell are all possibilities. In short, make your space your own and allow it to grow and flourish as you do.

Once you have made your home your own, treat it as sacred. Develop small rituals that you use to signal to yourself and to your guests that they're at your house. In traditional Russia, honored guests are greeted with a gift of bread and salt. In Hawaii, a lei of flowers or leaves is a traditional welcome. In Benin, I was once greeted by being offered a simple enameled basin filled with cool, fragrant water, which, casting aside all thoughts of cholera and malaria, I had to sip. When I asked about the custom, I was informed that the friend's mother whom we were visiting was from Niger, an arid country. There, the best possible gift that one could offer to a visitor was cool water—a magnificent thought.

I was so impressed by that welcoming sip of fragrant water that I asked what had perfumed the water. I was told that aromatic grasses are placed in jars of water and left to steep. They give the water a particular taste. In parts of Mexico, water jugs are made from a clay that imparts its special taste to the water.

You can create your own welcoming ritual. If you like the idea of cooling, refreshing water, why not try keeping a bottle of water in the refrigerator with lemon slices dotted with cloves in it. You may wish to experiment and invent a house drink. Mine was simple champagne. The first year that I was in my house, I made a point of serving all first-time visitors champagne in my amber champagne flutes. You could make yours Bloody Marys, kirs, anything from mulled cider in the winter to your own blend of iced herb tea in the summer—or simple fragrant water.

My friend June asks her friends to take off their shoes when they visit. When she has a party, there are rows of shoes lined up outside the door to her apartment. Small things make a difference, but they all signify a welcome to your space. Any gesture can be a welcome. I can't try to duplicate that.

A final note about your home environment: take time out to create your own special space within your home. Whether you are Roman Catholic, Buddhist, Muslim, Wiccan, Yoruba, or Moon Child, leave a spot for your faith in your home. It should be a place where you go to center yourself and find the energy that you have lost during the day, a place of peace and meditation and a place of tranquillity. You don't have to practice any religion actively to appreciate the difference in you that a special spot to meditate and find peace can create. A friend of mine who professes no specific faith has created her own ancestor altar in her home. It borrows from many faiths, but is full of photographs of deceased members of her family. When she is feeling low or in need of help, she heads there. She talks to her folks and feels at one with the continuity of her family. As she puts it, "All I have to do is think of the folks, tell them what I need, and it comes."

Your environment extends beyond your home to your car and even to your workplace. No matter how rigid your office's rules are, you can usually personalize your work space, perhaps with a picture or a funny calender. At my office, I was unlucky enough to lose the draw and be allotted a windowless office. When I first got into my four-walled box, I was in despair. The door was always open so that I could see life. I was unhappy about my office for about a year; then I realized that I was wrong—I had my own secret hideaway, away from all the outside madness. I brought in items from my collection of African and Brazilian art, hung a Haitian voodoo flag to the Marassa or twins on the wall, and got a funky cow calender, a French poster of horrible cat-related puns, and a poster of a big black Brazilian woman dancing frenetically. I added a naive-art pencil holder, brought in some fragrant potpourri, and am happy as a clam in my sanctuary with my door shut. I know that not everyone has the decorating flexibility in her office space that I do, but the point is the same: personalize and particularize. You have to work there and you should know that it's your space. If you can't put up anything or display personal items, make yourself a portable bag of talismans.

Talisman Tote
(For those who cannot particularize their spaces)

1 six-inch-square piece of your favorite fabric

1 feather you found on the street or the beach or in the woods

1 beach stone or pebble that appeals to you

4 other small items that have special meaning only to you

Fold the fabric in half and sew up two sides of it. Run a narrow hem around the open side and run a small cord through the hem to serve as a drawstring. Alternately, you can purchase a small draw-string bag in a fabric that you like. When the bag is ready, fill it with the items you have found or selected. Try to find items that appeal to all your senses. Carry the bag with you when you go to places that you cannot decorate. When you arrive, hang the bag on the back of your chair, or simply place it at your work space. You'll know that you're not anonymous and that some of what makes you, you is right there with you. No one has to know, but you'll feel better for it.

Two final notes about life enhancers: Allow time for yourself. We all get too busy to do what we truly enjoy. Some of us get so busy we actually forget what it is that we enjoy. Take time out for yourself. If it means taking a long walk after you come home from work, do it. If it means allowing time to read something for yourself before turning off the light at night, take the time to do it, even if it means you have to go to bed earlier or sacrifice a few minutes of sleep. Give yourself some time each day. The rest of the work will always get done.

Finally, it may come as a surprise to many of us, but attitude toward life means everything in terms of life expectancy. Even insurance actuarial tables take it into consideration. They suggest that a happy outlook toward life can go a long way toward keeping you healthy and alive. Think about it. Now isn't that the best life enhancer of all?

MAIL-ORDER RESOURCES

Herbal Supplies

Aphrodisia
264 Bleecker St.
New York, NY 10014
(212) 989-5440

Bay Laurel Farm
West Garzas Rd.
Carmel Valley, CA 93924
(408) 659-2913

Shepherd's Garden Seeds
6116 Highway 9
Felton, CA 95018
(408) 355-5311

May Way Trading
Chinese Herb Company
1338 Cypress St.
Oakland, CA 94607
(510) 208-3113

Wilton Organic Plants
357 Harlem and Catherine Avenues
Pasadena, MD 31122
(410) 647-1561

Tai Sang Trading
Chinese Herb Company
1018 Stockton
San Francisco, CA 94108
(415) 981-5364

Essential Oils

Caswell Massey Company, Ltd.
100 Enterprise Place
Dover, DE 19901
(800) 326-0500

Kiehl's Pharmacy
109 Third Ave.
New York, NY 10003
(212) 475-3400

Vineyard Sound Herbs
Vineyard Haven, MA 02557
(508) 696-7574

Other

Magikal Child
35 West 19th Street
New York, NY 10011
(212) 242-7182

Appendix B

SUGGESTED READING

Africa, Llaila O. *African Holistic Health.* N.P.: Adesegun, Johnson & Koram, 1989.

Angeloglou, Maggie. *A History of Makeup.* New York: Macmillan, 1970.

Baird, Mary A., and Keith E. Baird. *Sea Island Roots.* Trenton, NJ: Africa World, 1991.

Benedetti, María Delores Hajosy. *Hasta los baños te curan!* San Juan, Puerto Rico: Editorial Cultural, 1992.

Beuze, Renée. *La santé par les plantes des Antilles françaises.* Fort-de-France, Martinique: Desormeaux, 1973.

Brafford, C. J., and Liane Thom. *Dancing Colors.* San Francisco: Chronicle, 1992.

Budapest, Zsuzsanna E. *The Goddess in the Office.* San Francisco: HarperSanFrancisco, 1993.

Caron, Michel, and Henry Clos Jouve. *Plantas medicinales.* Barcelona: Daimon, 1966.

Densmore, Frances. *How Indians Use Wild Plants for Food, Medicine and Crafts.* New York: Dover, 1974.

Eliade, Mircea. *Gods, Goddesses, and Myths of Creation.* New York: Harper & Row, 1974.

Fraizer, Gregory, and Beverly Fraizer. *The Bath Book.* San Francisco: Troubador, 1973.

Hirschfelder, Arlene, and Paulette Molin. *The Encyclopedia of Native American Religions.* New York: Facts on File, 1992.

Honychurch, Penelope N. *Caribbean Wild Plants and Their Uses.* London: Macmillan/Caribbean, 1986.

Hubert-Schoumann, Annie. *La beauté par les plantes tropicales.* Fort-de-France, Martinique: Desormeaux, 1980.

Jahadhmy, Ali A. *Anthology of Swahili Poetry*. London: Heinemann, 1975.

Jordan, Portia Brown. *Herbal Medicine and Home Remedies: A Potpourri in Bahamian Culture*. Nassau: Guardian, 1986.

Khadraoui, Othman, ed. *Le hammam*. Tunis: Ceres, 1992.

Krakow, Amy. *The Total Tattoo Book*. New York: Warner, 1994.

Louis, Andre. *Le mariage traditionnel tunisien*. Sousse, Tunisia: C.R.B.D., 1990.

Lucas, Richard. *Secrets of the Chinese Herbalists*. West Nyack, NY: Parker, 1977.

Lund, Duane R. *Early Native American Recipes and Remedies*. Staples, MN: Lund, 1991.

Miller, Richard Alan, and Iona Miller. *The Magic and Ritual Use of Perfumes*. Rochester, VT: Destiny, 1990.

Mitchell, Faith. *Hoodoo Medicine*. San Francisco: Reed, Cannon & Johnson, 1978.

Morris, Edwin T. *Fragrance*. New York: Scribners, 1984.

Morton, Julia F. *Folk Remedies of the Low Country*. Miami: Seeman, 1974.

Ody, Penelope. *The Complete Medicinal Herbal*. London: Dorling Kindersley, 1993.

Richter, Anne. *Arts and Crafts of Indonesia*. San Francisco: Chronicle, 1994.

Robertson, Diane. *Live Longer, Look Younger with Herbs*. Kingston, Jamaica: Stationery & School Supplies, 1990.

Sagay, Esi. *African Hairstyles*. Oxford: Heinemann, 1983.

Smyth, Angela. *The Complete Home Healer*. San Francisco: HarperSanFrancisco, 1994.

Sun Bear, Wabun Wind, and Chrysalis Mulligan. *Dancing the Wheel*. New York: Fireside, 1992.

Teish, Luish. *Jambalaya*. San Francisco: Harper & Row, 1985.

Tisserand, Maggie. *Aromatherapy for Women*. Rochester, VT: Healing Arts, 1988.

———. *Essence of Love*. San Francisco: HarperSanFrancisco, 1993.

Wade, Carlson. *Health Secrets from the Orient*. New York: Signet, 1973.

Index

...oked and drained... and a splash of the reserved pasta water. Toss and add more pasta water if it seems a little dry. (I usually end up adding about 3/4 cup of pasta water.)

Serve the pasta with the burrata on top (if you're using it) and a generous drizzle of reduced balsamic vinegar.

CBD OIL

Ingredients:

7-10 grams of ground, dried cannabis
1 ½ cups of coconut oil
1/3 cup olive oil (optional)
1/3 cup beeswax
1 baking sheet
1 saucepan (or double boiler)
1 jar
1 cheesecloth
A few drops of essential oil (your choice)

Preheat your oven to 240 degrees Fahrenheit and spread your dried ground cannabis on a baking sheet.
When the oven is preheated, decarboxylate your cannabis in the oven for 25-30 minutes.
While your cannabis is in the oven, place your coconut and olive oil in the saucepan or double boiler over low heat and stir continuously.
Remove your decarboxylated cannabis from the oven and mix it into the coconut oil. Maintain a low heat and continue stirring the cannabis and oil mixture for 20 to 25 minutes.